The Botox Book

The Botox Book

**What You Need to Know
About America's Most Popular
Cosmetic Treatment**

Everett M. Lautin, M.D.,
and Suzanne M. Levine, D.P.M.,

and Kathryn Lance

M. Evans and Company, Inc. • New York

DISCLAIMER

This publication is designed to provide accurate and authoritative information in regard to the subject matter covered. It is sold with the understanding that the publisher is not engaged in rendering professional services. If legal, accounting, medical, psychological, or any other expert assistance is required, the services of a competent professional person should be sought.

The information, ideas, procedures, and suggestions contained in this book are not intended to replace the services of a trained health-care professional or to serve as a replacement for professional medical advice and care or as a substitute for any treatment prescribed by your physician. Matters regarding an individual's health often require medical supervision. A physician or health-care professional should be consulted regarding the use of any of the ideas, procedures, suggestions, or drug therapies in this book. Any application of the information set forth in this book is at the reader's discretion. The author and publisher hereby specifically disclaim any and all liability arising directly or indirectly from the use or application of any of the products, ideas, procedures, drug therapies, or suggestions contained in this book and any errors, omissions, and inaccuracies in the information contained herein.

Trade names are included for identification purposes only, and are not intended to endorse the product.

M. Evans and Company, Inc.
216 East 49th Street
New York, New York 10017

Library of Congress Cataloging-in-Publication Data

TK

Printed in the United States of America

9 8 7 6 5 4 3 2 1

I dedicate this book to my colleague and friend, Suzanne M. Levine, D.P.M., for her inspiration; my father, Arthur Lautkin, for teaching me the power of logical thinking; my mother, Fredda B. Lautkin, for her support; and my children, Douglas and Dana, for being there.

—Everett M. Lautin

I dedicate this book to my colleague and friend, Everett M. Lautin, M.D., for his intelligence and originality; and my children, Marissa and Heather, for their support.

—Suzanne M. Levine

Contents

Acknowledgments

We are grateful to all the beauty and fashion editors whose critical aesthetic skills and insights have proved invaluable in guiding and fine-tuning our aesthetic senses. In particular, we acknowledge Anna Wintour, Amy Astley, Jillian Demling, and André Talley of *Vogue* magazine; DiDi Gluck of *Marie Claire*; Sallie Brady of *Concord* magazine; and Gena Way of *US Weekly*. We also thank Katie Couric, Emiko Tate, and Betsy Alexandra of the *Today Show*; Florence Henderson of *Later Today*, and her beautiful daughter, Barbara Chase; Karen Harris of NBC news; Susan Ducher of NBC *Weekend Today Show*; Matt Strauss and Elena George (Emmy Award–winning makeup artist) at *The View*; High Voltage, who helped transform us; and Donna Lapkin, whose aesthetic sensibilities and courage guided us.

We acknowledge the untiring efforts of Kathryn Lance in providing background research and compiling this book in a thorough yet expeditious manner.

We acknowledge the consummate editing skills of PJ Dempsey and George de Kay of M. Evans and Company, Inc. for making this book possible.

We acknowledge our dedicated staff: Wincess Elias, Jinet Delgado, Louise Russo, Toni Lopez Morales, and Chloe.

And, of course, we acknowledge all of our wonderful patients who provided a beautiful canvas on which we could work.

Introduction

As doctors dedicated to making people look and feel better about themselves, we've worked for years to offer our patients the latest and most effective rejuvenation treatments and preparations. For more than four years, we've been proud to make available a number of treatments using Botox, which can truly be called a miracle drug.

Since the early nineties, Botox has been used with virtually 100 percent safety to relieve a number of medical conditions that were previously untreatable or had unsatisfactory treatments, including those associated with crossed eyes and painful muscle spasms. In the past few years, Botox has been found safe and effective to treat migraine headaches and even embarrassing sweating. Even more recently, spasms of the esophagus, tremors from stroke and cerebral palsy, and back pain have been added to the list. It seems as if almost every day a new use is found for Botox.

Among the most exciting uses of Botox are for improving or

even erasing the most obvious signs of aging. For example, those deep wrinkles and furrows that we refer to as laugh lines or frown lines can begin to appear even in those in their late twenties and thirties. Patients who have had Botox treatments for this purpose are uniformly thrilled with their new appearance. Botox can even improve one of the most unattractive signs of aging—the stringy "turkey neck" that appears in most people in their late forties to mid-fifties.

Until very recently, the only thing that could be done to rejuvenate an aging neck or facial wrinkles and furrows was surgery—a face-lift or brow-lift. We've all seen the results—a pulled-back, unnatural, wide-eyed appearance, not to mention the pain, expense, and downtime involved. Even worse, surgical procedures can damage the nerves to the face and compromise the blood supply, leading to uneven skin tone and an asymmetrical appearance. To add insult to injury, people who have had face lifts do not age gracefully—someone in her eighties who had a face-lift at age fifty often looks noticeably worse than someone who never had any cosmetic treatments at all.

Luckily for all the thirty- and forty-somethings, as well as the aging baby boomers who are patients at our Manhattan office, Institute Beauté, nature herself has come to the rescue. Though it is much more than a miracle wrinkle cure, Botox allows us to help our patients age gracefully while looking their best—and yes, looking younger. With virtually no significant side effects and no recovery time, the safety of Botox is unparalleled, which is why, on April 15, 2002, the Food and Drug Administration (FDA) approved the use of Botox specifically for the cosmetic treatment of frown furrows above the nose between the eyebrows.

Like many other doctors, we've used Botox off-label for several years—that is, although Botox had been originally approved only for certain medical uses involving muscle spasms, we've used it for a number of cosmetic purposes as well. Off-label use is a common and legal practice with many drugs, especially new ones for which new uses are still being discovered.

We've had overwhelming acceptance by our patients. In fact, satisfaction with Botox is among the highest of all the many procedures and treatments that we offer. As experience with this wonder drug grows, researchers continue to find new uses for it. In addition, new variants of Botox-like drugs are being developed.

Is Botox right for you? What exactly is it, and how does it work? What medical conditions and cosmetic problems can it treat? We hope to answer all these questions and more in the next few chapters.

Chapter 1
What Is Botox?

You have probably heard about botulism, a type of food poisoning caused by one of the most deadly toxins known. You surely remember warnings not to eat food from a bulging can, or home-canned products that haven't been cooked long enough. Those are the most common ways to contract botulism, though it can be spread through other kinds of food as well.

Although most cases of botulism are caused by improperly preserved food, there are other kinds of botulism poisoning, including one that infects wounds and another that makes very young babies sick. There are also types of botulism that only affect particular animals such as birds.

All types of botulism are caused by the bacterium *Clostridium botulinum*, which can live for a very long time as a spore, the reproductive stage of certain bacteria and fungi. When botulinum spores are placed in a moist, low-acid environment without oxygen (such as inside a can of improperly canned food), they begin to grow into mature bacteria and give off their deadly toxin, botulinum. There are actually nine different types of botulinum toxin. The two that are currently used medically are Botulinum A and Botulinum B.

Harnessing a Deadly Poison

Botulinum toxin is considered a *neurotoxin*, which means that it interferes with the function of the nervous system. Other neurotoxins include scorpion venom, some snake venoms, some pesticides, and many other natural and synthetic compounds. Neurotoxins are among the most deadly of all poisons.

Botulinum toxin works primarily by disrupting the communication between nerves and the muscles they control, though it can also affect other nerve functions. It enters the nerve ending and blocks the release of an important neurochemical, *acetylcholine*, which signals muscles to contract. Without this chemical message, the muscle responds to nerve signals only very feebly or not at all. In other words, it becomes very weak or paralyzed.

When people have been poisoned by botulism, all their major muscles gradually become paralyzed, and, if the dose is high enough and they don't receive supportive therapy (which may include respiratory support, intravenous fluids, tube feedings, and skilled nursing care), they become unable to breathe and die of suffocation. However, with proper therapy, the nerves repair themselves, sprouting new endings and reestablishing the nerve–muscle connections. About twenty years ago, scientists figured out how to take botulism's deadly ability—to paralyze muscles—and harness it to cure ailments such as spasms that are caused by overactive muscles.

The botulinum toxin used for medical purposes has been refined and purified, and is used only in very tiny amounts, on specific muscles, rather than throughout the body. These amounts are so small that there is virtually no danger of systemic side effects (side effects that involve the whole body). In approximately three to five months, depending on where the Botox has been injected, and for what purpose, the effect gradually wears off and new injections must be given.

Where It Came From

Botulinum toxin was first used for medical purposes in humans in the late 1980s as a treatment for certain neurological disorders. A highly purified form of the strongest toxin, Botulinum A, was eventually developed as Botox for patients suffering from eyelid spasms and misaligned (crossed) eyes. By weakening the muscle responsible for the difficulty, Botox temporarily improved the condition. It was officially approved for this use by the FDA in December 1989 and approved for relaxing neck spasms a year later.

In the late 1980s, Alastair and Jean Carruthers, a husband-and-wife doctor team in Vancouver, Canada, compared notes and made an amazing discovery: the wrinkles that Alastair, a dermatologist, had been treating with collagen injections were easily erased by the use of Botox, which Jean had been using as an ophthalmologist to treat eyelid spasms. In addition to improving the eye condition, the Botox had also weakened the muscles that caused frown lines and crow's feet, leading her patients to look younger and more relaxed.

Experimenting on their receptionist and themselves, the Carruthers demonstrated to their own satisfaction that Botox was actually superior to collagen injections in producing a more rested and youthful facial appearance. Thus was born the most important medical cosmetic advance in decades. Throughout the 1990s, plastic surgeons, dermatologists, and other doctors began to use Botox on their patients who were bothered by lines on their foreheads and around their eyes. These lines (dynamic wrinkles), which are caused mainly by overactive muscles, can make you look tired, or angry, or older than you are. A lot of people habitually squint or frown without being aware of it, and over time the lines become etched into the face. But when the involved muscles become weakened, the lines start to disappear.

The results of using Botox to control unwanted facial lines were so promising that patients told their friends about this new treatment. These friends told their friends and so on. By 2000, over one million people had been treated with Botox.

According to the American Society of Plastic Surgeons, Botox is now the most popular nonsurgical cosmetic procedure in the United States. The American Society for Aesthetic Plastic Surgery, an advocacy group for plastic surgeons, reports that more than 1.5 million Botox procedures were performed in 2001, mostly on women in the thirty-five- to fifty-year-old age bracket. We find in our practice that Botox is one of the most often requested treatments, and one of the most successful, according to the enthusiastic comments of satisfied patients.

FDA Approval for Cosmetic Use

Because Botox was so effective in the muscle-related medical problems that it was originally used for, doctors began to use it off-label in the 1990s to treat other conditions involving muscles. This is a perfectly legal process that occurs with many promising drugs and often leads to new cures for a variety of ailments.

Since then, thousands of doctors and millions of patients have proven Botox's effectiveness in a variety of medical and cosmetic procedures. In a series of scientifically controlled clinical trials, researchers conclusively demonstrated that Botox reduces the frown lines between the eyes. In April 2002, the FDA approved Botox for this use. It is expected to approve the drug for crow's feet and forehead wrinkles soon.

The approval of the FDA means not only that patients can count on the efficacy and safety of Botox; it also means that Botox will become more widely available and costs may come down. The approval allows the manufacturer of Botox, Allergan, to advertise Botox for the specific purpose for which it has been accepted. As a result, Allergan is promoting the drug as a treatment for frown lines under the name Cosmetic Botox. The strength, purity, and cost of Cosmetic Botox are the same as Botox used for medical purposes; only the label is different.

Safety

Unlike many trendy new drugs, Botox has been thoroughly tested for safety. Although it is always possible with any drug of natural origin for an allergic reaction to develop, so far there have been no reports of systemic (body-wide) reactions from the many uses of Botox.

How can a toxin so dangerous be made so safe? The answer is in the size of the dose. Botox is packaged in vials that each contain 100 units of the drug. The number of units that would be needed to kill someone is estimated to be thirty-five times that amount—3,000 to 3,500 units, or thirty to thirty-five vials. An average cosmetic treatment with Botox, in contrast, requires much less than one full vial—only about 30 units of the toxin, or one-one hundredth of a lethal dose. More extensive procedures, such as those required to relax the neck muscles, still use a relatively small amount, 50 to 100 units, or for hyperhidrosis (excessive sweating) treatment, 200 to 300 units, which also leaves a very large margin of safety.

There are some side effects to Botox, depending on where in the body it is used. The most common problems occur in the face and neck, especially with medical uses of the drug, which require a larger dose. The side effects that appear most often are a drooping eyelid or eyebrow when Botox is used in this area, and, rarely, difficulty in swallowing when Botox is used in the neck. These problems clear up on their own without treatment, usually in a few weeks or less. An experimental antidote is being developed based on human antibodies that can block these effects.

The biggest drawback to using Botox is that a small percentage of patients (fewer than 5 percent) develop antibodies to the toxin. Instead of causing an allergic reaction, these antibodies prevent the toxin from working. This reaction is most likely in those who use relatively large amounts, such as people who are receiving Botox for muscle spasms. A different form of botulinum toxin (Botulinum B), marketed under the name Myobloc by Elan Pharmaceuticals, may work on people who have developed antibodies to Botulinum A (see chapter 4 for more on Myobloc).

To further ensure safety, Allergan, the manufacturer, recommends that Botox should be injected only once every three months, using the lowest possible effective dosage. Botox must be administered by a physician, although some states allow for the drug to be administered by nurse practitioners. Our opinion is that Botox should always be injected under a physician's supervision.

Is There a Downside to Botox?

It's hard to believe that something once considered a public health menace has become one of the most effective and trusted medications used by doctors of many specialties. Even more amazing is that the same medication is a safe and potent facial rejuvenator. So what, you may ask, do some people view as the downside?

- **Botox can have annoying and even serious side effects.** While any drug can have side effects, with Botox the annoying ones are uncommon and the serious ones are rare, but are more likely to occur when Botox is administered by inexperienced or unqualified practitioners. These effects include muscular weakness, drooping eyelids, and difficulty in swallowing (depending on the area treated). However, these effects are rare and will disappear of their own accord in a few days to a few weeks. For more details on the possible side effects of Botox, see the sections on specific procedures.

- **Some people don't respond to Botox or stop responding after several injections.** It is true that a small number of people (3 to 5 percent) don't respond to Botox injections and that a slightly larger percentage stop responding after a series of successful treatments. A different form of botulinum toxin, marketed under the name Myobloc, appears to work on many people who have developed Botox resistance. To learn more about

Myobloc and other variants of the toxin under development, see chapter 4.

- **The cost of continuing treatments is prohibitive.**
The fact is that Botox treatments need to be repeated indefinitely to maintain their effects. For many medical procedures, this isn't a problem, since insurance companies are beginning to routinely cover such treatments. Cosmetic treatments are not covered, however, and their continuing cost could be a problem for some patients.

  But as Botox continues to gain in popularity, costs per treatment should go down somewhat. Also, there is evidence that in many patients the effect of treatments might last longer with repeated use. Compared to more expensive rejuvenation procedures, such as deep peels or plastic surgery, Botox is a bargain. As one of our patients says, "I don't mind paying for it. It's part of my upkeep, like getting my hair cut and colored."

  For more information on Botox costs, see the cost guidelines in chapter 5.

- **Botox turns you into an expressionless zombie.**
No one denies that inaccurate injections of either too much Botox or Botox in the wrong place can give an expressionless, mask-like appearance to the face. But this should not happen if the procedure is done by an experienced practitioner, who will inject enough toxin to relax your lines or wrinkles but not enough to totally paralyze an area of your face. Remember, too, that Botox is forgiving, in that its

effects are temporary.

Obviously, you should make sure that your doctor is experienced. In an interview in Newsweek, Dr. Ezra Kest, a Beverly Hills dermatologist who routinely treats actors, emphasizes that "if you do the injections the proper way, you can give them [patients] a natural expression without the little lines."

- **People should just accept that they're getting older and age gracefully.** We respect the decision of men and women who wish to look older as they grow older. That is certainly their right. But those who want to continue to look younger—whether for career reasons or just because it makes them feel better about themselves—also have the right to choose Botox or other treatments.

Dr. Alicia Farr, a veterinarian in San Diego, California, had Botox injections for a deep furrow between her eyebrows a year ago, when she was fifty-nine. "The wrinkle was so deep I could stick my thumbnail into it," she says. "I didn't want it there." She also didn't want forehead wrinkles, and injections of Botox took care of that problem too. Now, Dr. Farr says, most people tell her that she looks about fifty. "Some people are old at thirty," she says. "A generation ago, they were old at my age. But I'm not ready for the rocking chair. I take care of myself and I have a lot of energy. Looking younger makes me feel better about myself."

The bottom line, as far as we're concerned, is why look older than you have to? With little risk, little pain, and no downtime, Botox makes it easy to continue to look your best.

Chapter 2
Everybody's Doing It

Today, it seems as if the whole world has heard of Botox. It's one of the most popular cosmetic treatments on the planet: physicians are offering injections in Europe, the Middle East, Japan, Australia, Mexico, and South America. Botox clinics do a thriving business in nearly all first-world countries and even some developing countries. According to the *Times of India,* in 2001 a day-long workshop in Bangalore was organized by the Cosmetology Society of India to brief doctors on the benefits of this miracle drug.

Unlike more traditional cosmetic treatments, especially plastic surgery, patients are coming in at younger and younger ages. While the latest figures show that the majority of patients for all cosmetic treatments are in the forty- to fifty-nine-year-old age range, a growing number—nearly a third—are in their twenties and thirties. Botox has added to this trend because its effects are subtle and almost immediate, and because there is evidence that early use helps prevent worsening of many of the signs of aging.

Among the first people to use Botox regularly were those who had to because their jobs demanded that they look their best at all times: models, movie actors and actresses, and television personalities. From these few pioneers the practice has grown to where, rumor has it, present-day news and entertainment anchors must be willing to undergo Botox and other treatments in order to get a contract.

Although there's no doubt that Botox is currently used by many prominent Hollywood and television personalities, most still decline to reveal that their good looks are partly due to Botox. Speaking in *USA Today*, Dr. Nasreen Babu-Khan, a dermatologist and associate clinical professor of medicine at the University of Southern California, notes that "celebrities don't really want anyone to know how they keep themselves looking so good." Among those who have admitted to receiving Botox treatments, even recommending it to others, are Madonna, Carrie Fisher, Joan Rivers, and Annie Potts. Botox is so popular among the Hollywood set, in fact, that one Beverly Hills clinic reportedly offers pre-Oscar treatments for half price. Another more credible rumor maintains that Oscar-bound starlets get Botox treatments in their armpits before the ceremony to prevent the telltale nervous sign of sweating (and to preserve those expensive rented gowns).

It makes sense that people in the public eye would want to do whatever it takes to look their best; the truth is that better looks can actually be an advantage for most of us. A number of research studies have been done on the connection between attractiveness and job promotions or pay. Dr. Daniel Hamermesh, an economist at the University of Texas at Austin and the author of several papers on the connection between beauty and job success, has found that in several countries, including the United States, there is a pay premium of up to 5 percent for being very attractive. Likewise, people perceived as having below-average looks make up to 10 percent less money than their average-looking counter-parts.

Dr. Hamermesh is quick to caution that higher earnings are only one of many reasons why people might spend money on treatments such as Botox. "Actually," he says, "my work on Chinese women and beauty treatments suggests that most of the money spent on beautification does not pay off in higher earnings later on." Still, the correlation between higher pay and better looks holds true for both men and women, which may explain why so many men are getting Botox and other rejuvenation treatments.

The American Society of Plastic Surgeons has published statistics showing that approximately 88 percent of Botox procedures are currently performed on women, but men make up a growing minority of those receiving the treatments—as high as 20 percent according to some doctors. In our practice, at Institute Beauté, approximately 15 percent of our Botox patients are men.

One group of men who use Botox in growing numbers are trial lawyers. According to the *Wall Street Journal,* some top male attorneys receive Botox treatments prior to facing a jury so that they will appear more sympathetic and less angry. A study conducted by Dr. Hamermesh and colleagues showed that lawyers rated as good-looking at the start of law school generally achieved overall higher earnings than their less attractive colleagues.

Citing earlier studies, Dr. Hamermesh speculates that since people have been shown to find attractive communicators more persuasive than unattractive ones, "An attorney who is better able to persuade and convince others, particularly judges and juries, may be producing higher-quality legal services."

Looking better is not just about earnings; it can markedly impact other important areas of your life. For example, improving your appearance can also improve your self-esteem, and, if you're among the growing number of middle-aged divorceés, it can help you feel more competitive in the dating arena.

Not everyone can be strikingly beautiful or handsome, of course. But most of us have it within our power to improve our general looks, and this is especially true when it comes to signs of aging. As Dr. Hamermesh points out, while it's true that you can't make a silk purse out of a sow's ear, "the sow's ear's appeal can be improved upon somewhat."

For all of these reasons—better job prospects, stronger self-esteem, and improved interpersonal relations—the use of Botox for cosmetic purposes has moved beyond the rich, famous, and well connected. Today, it is rapidly gaining acceptance among ordinary people: housewives, teachers, business executives—in short, anyone who wants to look his or her best, for whatever reason and no matter how old.

As one of our patients said, looking into the mirror after a recent treatment, "When I used to look at myself, I'd see all the little flaws—things other people didn't notice. Now I look so much better that I'm much less critical of myself."

Botox Parties

Because Botox is expensive and must be used quickly after it has been prepared (it has a shelf life of approximately twenty-four hours in the refrigerator), friends sometimes have treatments at the same time to share a vial of the toxin and prevent it from going to waste. We, along with many other doctors, have begun to organize such sharing as a way to provide the treatments more economically.

"Botox parties," said to have started among London socialites, have become the rage. At these gatherings, women (and some men) meet to socialize and share treatments of Botox at their local dermatology office or beauty spa—or even in someone's home, with one room temporarily converted into a rejuvenation clinic.

We think Botox parties are a great idea provided that the treatments are administered by an experienced physician. At the most recent Botox party put on by Institute Beauté, the newly revitalized guests left feeling better and thinking that they looked better, and in a few days they will.

Don't think that Botox parties are just for the upper crust or those lucky enough to live in major cities. One plastic surgeon in Florida has even begun hosting Botox "happy hours" for the suburban after-work set. Typically, Botox parties include drinks and snacks in a relaxed setting, combined with a physician's services. Treatments may be discounted, and the event will probably include a discussion or lecture on the benefits and risks of using Botox.

Mixing beautification with wine and hors d'oeuvres may sound like a winning combination, but before you opt for Botox and Beaujolais, check out the setting and the physician to make sure that both are on the up and up. And go easy on the wine—alcohol before any medical procedure can increase the risk of bleeding, and in the case of Botox, bruising.

Ask these questions before you RSVP to a Botox party:

- **Is the physician experienced with the cosmetic use of Botox and board certified?** (For further tips on choosing a doctor, see chapter 9).

- **Is the setting hygienic?** A doctor's office may not seem as glamorous as a spa, but it is a much safer setting for what is, after all, a medical procedure.

- **Is the Botox fresh and not overdiluted?**

- **Has the physician allotted sufficient time to thoroughly discuss the procedure with each patient?** For questions you should discuss before treatment, see chapter 9.

Chapter 3
What It Does and
How It Works

It's strange to think of a toxin that affects muscles as a wrinkle cure. But it makes perfect sense once you understand what really causes wrinkles and how Botox works. Basically, there are two types of wrinkles. *Dynamic wrinkles,* or muscle wrinkles, form where muscles move the face the most (around and between the eyes and around the mouth). *Static wrinkles* are lines and crinkles that appear at the corners of the eyes and in other areas on the face. Because it affects the facial muscles, Botox can help ease or prevent both types.

Dynamic wrinkles go deep. As they develop, they create actual furrows in the skin, like ditches in a landscape. Their appearance is obvious even when you're not moving a muscle in your face. Before Botox, the only safe and natural-looking way to fully erase a dynamic wrinkle was to literally fill it in with injectable implants such as collagen, and that's still helpful in a number of cases.

Static wrinkles are more superficial and tend to appear most obviously when the face is moving, such as when you smile or frown. These are the fine lines and crinkles that can give your age away even if the rest of your face is smooth. There are a number of ways to help minimize or eliminate these wrinkles, and one of the best is by using Botox.

Both types of lines appear because all of us habitually scowl or squint, eventually forming permanent lines and crinkles in the skin. Unlike other treatments that fill in the wrinkle, or strip away the top layer of skin along with the wrinkle, Botox actually goes to the source of the wrinkle by preventing the squinting or scowling in the first place.

Imagine that your skin is a bed sheet with two people pulling on opposite corners, creating a diagonal furrow in the sheet. Now, if both people drop the sheet, you can simply smooth it out, eliminating the furrow and the associated smaller wrinkles. That's something like what happens with Botox. A minute amount of the poison is injected, which weakens or paralyzes the muscles pulling on the skin by blocking the chemical that causes them to contract. This allows the muscles to relax and in turn lets the skin smooth out over the facial structure.

Once Botox is injected into a muscle, the muscle will lose much of its strength and simply be unable to pull on the skin. Over time, the existing wrinkles will begin to disappear, as if someone had smoothed them over. When your face is at rest, the furrows will not be visible; when you frown, they will not be so deep.

It's important to make sure that too much Botox is not injected, or the facial muscles won't move at all and your face will become expressionless. Be sure to choose a doctor with the experience and aesthetic sense to inject the appropriate dose of Botox for your particular situation. (For more on choosing a doctor, see chapter 9.)

So far, most Botox injections given for cosmetic reasons have been applied to the forehead and the area around the eyes. However, we and other doctors are increasingly using Botox to improve the appearance of lines around the mouth and from the mouth to the chin. This use is somewhat trickier and requires a very experienced physician in order to avoid interfering with movement of the lower face.

Another very exciting and growing use for Botox is in relaxing the platysma muscles of the neck, which separate into stringy lines with age, causing the ugly "turkey neck" effect. When those muscles are treated with Botox, the stringiness disappears along with horizontal lines, and the neck begins to resume a more youthful appearance.

Another effect of using Botox on the neck is an improved jaw-line, because the same platysma muscles that cause stringiness also pull down on the lower part of the face, accentuating the look of jowls and vertical lines. Although these signs of aging cannot be eliminated by Botox, in many people they are softened, resulting in a firmer and better-defined jawline.

The best thing about using Botox to erase wrinkles, besides its quick results and lack of downtime, is that it affects only the facial muscles injected directly. You will still be able to smile, laugh, and even show displeasure—but without the wrinkle-producing side effects.

Botox as a Preventive

We and many other physicians have noticed that for most Botox procedures the effects of each subsequent treatment tend to last longer before a new treatment is necessary. It's not known why this occurs. One possibility is that the involved muscles become permanently weakened by repeated applications of Botox; another is that they have become retrained. For example, if you are unable to scowl easily, as would be the case with Botox treatments to the forehead, you may simply stop trying to do so.

One of our patients, a fashion designer, began using Botox for her brow furrow and forehead wrinkles more than ten years ago (with another doctor). Now in her early fifties, Lorena is happier than ever with her relaxed appearance and notes that she needs the injections less frequently. "The crease between my eyes had been there since I was a teenager," she told us. "But the last time I needed an injection for it was two years ago. As for the forehead lines, I've noticed that I need fewer injections when I come in— they're spaced farther apart and I don't have to do them so often."

Because the cosmetic use of Botox is still relatively new, there are no long-term studies, but based on our patients' experience, we believe along with many other doctors that regular use of the drug earlier in life may indefinitely postpone some of the most obvious signs of aging, among them forehead furrows, crow's feet, and stringy turkey neck.

Who It's Good For

At Institute Beauté, we've used Botox to treat patients literally of all ages, from the early twenties to the late eighties. Results have been excellent in all age groups, though they are most dramatic in those whose signs of aging are still only minimal.

Although Botox can't restore the full blush of youth, it can make a big difference even in midlife or later. Ellen, a new patient who admits to being nearly sixty, had never previously considered any form of rejuvenation. A ghostwriter, Ellen had labored for years at home writing in relative obscurity, and, as she said, "not really caring what I looked like." All that changed when one of Ellen's own stories won an important award. The first time she saw her photograph in a national magazine, she was appalled. "It was huge," she said. "It showed everything. I hated it."

A friend recommended Institute Beauté. When we met Ellen,

we saw a pleasant woman who, while attractive, definitely looked her age. We explained her options, and Ellen opted for conservative treatment, mostly using Botox. "I don't care if I look younger," she told us. "I just don't want to look baggy, saggy, and haggy." Today Ellen looks younger and a lot more rested and attractive—and she feels better about herself.

Dr. Malcolm Paul, the president of the American Society for Aesthetic Plastic Surgery (ASAPS), which represents plastic surgeons in the United States and Canada, feels that Botox is one of the best treatments possible for people who won't consider plastic surgery or more drastic cosmetic treatments. Writing for the ASAPS web site, Dr. Paul states that "as a quick and effective treatment, with excellent results and virtually no downtime, it's perfect for those patients who have minimal signs of facial aging." He also recommends Botox for patients who show early signs of aging or who might not be good candidates for more traditional facial aesthetic surgery.

Although the use of Botox for a variety of cosmetic conditions is growing, at present we recommend it for patients who

- Have facial or neck wrinkles
- Are in good physical and emotional health
- Are motivated to improve their appearance
- Have realistic expectations
- Don't use recreational drugs
- Don't drink or smoke heavily

Contraindications

Although Botox is suitable for most people, its safety hasn't been established for women who are pregnant or breastfeeding. Because it affects the nervous system, its cosmetic use is not recommended for anyone with a neurological disorder, such as multiple sclerosis or Parkinson's disease. However, it can be used medically to treat some of the most troubling symptoms of these and other diseases (for more information, see chapter 4).

Other Botulinum Toxins

Botox is made from Botulinum A by Allergan and is currently the most popular and widely available preparation using botulinum toxin. At present it is also the only one approved by the FDA for both medical and cosmetic uses. A similar medication, Dysport, also made from Botulinum A, is available in Europe from Speywood Pharmaceuticals. The toxins are similar in their use and effects, but Botox is prepared in a stronger concentration.

The newest botulinum toxin available commercially is Myobloc, manufactured by Elan Pharmaceuticals. First introduced in January 2001, Myobloc is made from Botulinum B. The main advantage of Myobloc is that it is manufactured as a liquid, so it doesn't need to be mixed just before being used, as is the case with Botox, which comes freeze-dried and must be mixed with sterile, preservative-free, normal saline. It is also much more stable than Botox. Whereas Botox must be kept refrigerated and used within twenty-four hours of being mixed with saline solution, Myobloc can be kept at room temperature for as long as nine months, or refrigerated for two and a half years.

This long-term stability not only makes Myobloc much more convenient for physicians to use but makes it potentially less costly for patients. So far, Myobloc has only been approved by the FDA for neck spasms, but it is being used off-label for other medical conditions and cosmetic procedures.

Although Myobloc has not been as extensively studied as Botox, its effects are considered to be very similar, but it is not necessarily interchangeable with Botox in all cases. The safety record for Myobloc is considered to be comparable to that of Botox.

Clinical tests indicate that Myobloc may spread less to adjacent muscles than Botox. It is also somewhat faster-acting than Botox, producing results within one to two days rather than two to five days. There is conflicting evidence on how long Myobloc injections last. For some cosmetic procedures, it may not be quite as long-lasting as Botox, but it appears to last longer for certain medical uses, such as in relaxing neck spasms.

Because the two toxins are different in their chemical makeup, they can complement each other in certain ways. For example, Myobloc should work for the occasional patient who develops a resistance to Botox after many repeated injections. We've used Myobloc at Institute Beauté for all procedures for which we have used Botox, including for combating hyperhidrosis (excessive sweating), and have obtained very good results.

Researchers are currently investigating the seven other types of botulinum toxin. It is likely that several of them will be developed in the future for even more medical uses, and it is probable that bioengineered toxins will eventually be developed as well.

WHY I USE MYOBLOC
BY JASON N. POZNER, M.D., F.A.C.S.

In my plastic surgery practice in Florida, I use both Botox and Myobloc, and I find that Myobloc has some distinct advantages. For one thing, since it comes as a liquid and has a long refrigerated shelf life, you are always guaranteed to have fresh Myobloc on hand. The other advantage Myobloc has is its quick action. Most people have results within twelve hours of use, as opposed to three or four days for Botox.

This quick action can be a real advantage in some cases. Jennifer and Steve were a lovely couple in their early thirties getting married on Saturday at a posh Boca Raton country club. They hired the best wedding photographer in South Florida and had their families flying in from New York. However, Jennifer noticed some eye wrinkles when she smiled that looked terrible in her prewedding photographs. She'd had Botox before and wanted a quick fix before her big day.

Unfortunately, she came to see me on Thursday. "I know Botox usually takes a few days to work," she said, "but isn't there anything you can do to speed it up?"

I told her that there was no way to speed up Botox's action but advised her that Myobloc might solve her problem. I also warned that occasionally, as with Botox, you can get a bruise from the injection. She understood but wanted the injection, so I gave her the treatment.

I'm happy to say that Jennifer called the following Monday before leaving on her honeymoon to tell me that the Myobloc had worked perfectly and her wedding was a huge success. "And by the way," she added, "my mother wants an appointment as soon as possible."

Myobloc is not perfect, and I am sure it won't replace Botox anytime soon, because it doesn't seem to last as long as Botox for most procedures. As the price is comparable, unless Elan Pharmaceuticals finds a way to make Myobloc last longer, we will probably use Myobloc mainly for patients who have developed a resistance to Botox or for those who need its quick action.

WHAT BOTOX CAN AND CAN'T DO

WHAT BOTOX CAN DO:

- Relax tight or spastic muscles

- Smooth out wrinkles caused by muscle tension

- Smooth out wrinkles caused by muscle action

- Soften but not eliminate many signs of aging, including sagging

WHAT BOTOX CAN'T DO

- Improve skin texture

- Eliminate spots and blotches

- Rejuvenate collagen and elastin

- Tighten skin or eliminate sagging

Chapter 4
Medical Uses of Botox

Botox was originally used to improve two eye conditions caused by uneven or overactive eye muscles, and its medical uses have increased dramatically. Physicians are finding it effective in a wide variety of conditions that involve muscle spasms or tightening. The list is still growing, but among the ailments for which Botox offers new hope are facial tics, lower back pain, excessive sweating, and even stuttering.

Botox is so well established medically that insurance companies will now cover many uses related to muscles spasms or tightness. Check with your insurance company to see if preapproval is required. If you have problems getting reimbursed, Allergan, the maker of Botox, offers a program called the Botox Advantage, which aids patients with certain conditions in receiving insurance reimbursement for their treatments. For information, go to the Dystonia Foundation web site listed in Appendix A.

Achalasia (Spasms of the Esophagus)

One of the newest medical uses for Botox is in the treatment of *achalasia*, which is a disorder of the esophagus (food tube) characterized by difficulty in swallowing. This condition has many causes, but in all cases it results because the muscles of the esophagus no longer function properly, and spasms in the lower part of the esophagus make it difficult for food to pass into the stomach.

Before Botox, the only treatments for achalasia were medications, manual widening of the bottom of the esophagus, and surgery. The medications are effective for some people but have side effects ranging from headaches to low blood pressure. Manual widening of the bottom of the esophagus is done by inserting a tube containing a balloon into the esophagus, then inflating the balloon. This procedure is effective in a large number of patients but can also lead to rupture of the esophagus.

Surgical treatment for achalasia, called a myotomy, involves making a cut in the muscle of the lower esophagus, forcing it to relax. Myotomy is very effective, but hospitalization is required because the chest must be opened, there is a small risk of death during the procedure, and many patients have problems with acid reflux (GERD) afterward.

Botox treatment, which is performed through an endoscope (a slender fiber-optic tube that is inserted through the mouth into the esophagus), has also been very successful with a large number of patients. The main drawbacks are that it usually has to be repeated within a year and that patients may experience some chest pain immediately after the procedure. Because it is more difficult to perform a myotomy on patients who have already had Botox injections for this condition, some doctors recommend that Botox be used only on patients who are not suitable candidates for surgery.

Athlete's Foot

You don't have to be an athlete to get athlete's foot, although the fungus that causes this annoying condition thrives in the warm, moist conditions of a locker room. *Warm* and *moist* are the keywords, in fact, and explain why athlete's foot is so hard to get rid of once it has started. If you are very active and your feet sweat a lot, you're setting up a perfect incubator for foot fungus inside your shoes and on your feet.

Sweaty feet don't have to lead to a lifetime of itchy, red toes, however. By treating the excessive sweating with Botox, you eliminate one of the key conditions the fungus needs to live. For more details, read the section on hyperhidrosis.

Back Pain

Nearly 90 percent of adults experience back pain at some point in their lives. A significant number of people suffer for years, and there has been little medicine can do to alleviate their discomfort. Muscle relaxants, pain pills, and surgery have been the mainstay treatments until now. Not only do these treatments have side effects, but much of the time they don't even work. It's too early to say that Botox has provided the definitive cure for low back pain, but a recent study has given promising results: more than half the patients experienced relief from their pain, and there were no side effects. On average, the pain relief lasted four months until the Botox injections had to be repeated.

Blepharospasm (Eyelid Spasms)

Blepharospasm, uncontrolled blinking or spasms of the eyelid, was one of the first conditions for which Botox was approved by the FDA (in 1991). It can range from annoying to seriously debilitating. In severe cases, the eyelids can remain tightly closed for minutes to hours at a time. The eye itself remains healthy, but the patient becomes essentially blind.

This condition can have many causes, ranging from dry eyes to reactions to certain drugs. There was no really good treatment before Botox. A number of drugs were used, from muscle relaxants to antiseizure medications, but they had unpredictable side effects and didn't work on everybody. Surgical treatment, which involves removing some of the muscles of the eyelid, helps restore sight to many patients but can have unpleasant side effects, including blurred or double vision.

Since trials began in the late 1980s, Botox injections have been recognized as the best treatment for blepharospasm. The toxin relaxes the eye muscle, preventing spasms but allowing normal blinking. Some patients experience temporary side effects, including drooping eyelids, eye dryness, and double or blurred vision. As with all medical uses of Botox, the injections generally have to be repeated every few months.

For a small number of blepharospasm patients, the side effects remain bothersome. An experimental countertreatment has been developed using human botox immunoglobulin, which is a kind of antitoxin developed from human immune cells. It seems to reduce the side effects for blepharospasm patients and may be further developed to help in other conditions where the side effects of Botox are a problem.

Cerebral Palsy

Cerebral palsy, caused by brain injury at birth, can be character-ized by a number of problems ranging from difficulty in per-forming fine motor tasks (such as using scissors) to more serious disabilities ranging from retardation to inability to walk. Common muscle problems due to cerebral palsy are tremors, tics, and spasms of the muscles. In the past, these have been treated with various drugs and surgery, which have side effects and are not always successful.

Botox injections into the affected muscles have been very helpful in reducing or eliminating spasticity and tremors. As a rule, the first two series of injections are given every three months, with follow-up injections every six to nine months. Most insurance companies cover the injections.

Dysphonia (Vocal Cord Spasms)

This condition, technically known as dysphonia, is a form of dys-tonia (see below) affecting the vocal cords. Victims have difficul-ty talking, and their voice often sounds quivery or hoarse or dis-appears altogether. Before Botox, the few treatment options included cutting one of the nerves to the vocal cords (the symp-toms usually returned afterward), speech therapy, and psycho-logical counseling to help deal with the problem.

Botox therapy, consisting of repeated injections into the vocal cords, is very effective for most patients with this condition. In fact, 80 to 100 percent of people treated with Botox note a marked improvement. Possible side effects include occasional difficulty in swallowing and a breathy-sounding voice. In some patients the Botox stops working, but it is possible that these people can be helped by switching to injections of Myobloc (see chapter 3).

Dystonia (Muscle Spasms)

Dystonia is a condition in which the muscles go into involuntary spasms for unknown reasons. When the condition becomes chronic, it can cause great pain and serious problems. Blepharospasm is a form of dystonia affecting the eyelid muscles.

One of the earliest uses for Botox was in treating dystonia of the neck muscles, a painful and disabling condition in which the tight muscles force the head to one side. Although a number of drugs have been used to help patients with neck spasms, there was no good treatment for the condition, also known as torticollis or wry neck, until researchers began using Botox. The FDA approved Botox for this purpose in 1990.

Though it is most common in the eyelid and neck muscles, dystonia can affect other muscles in the body, including those in the arms, legs, and face. Botox has proven effective in helping to relax those muscles and relieve the condition. Ongoing research is studying the use of Botox for other kinds of dystonia.

Hyperhidrosis (Excessive Sweating)

Hyperhidrosis, or excessive sweating, is a very embarrassing and even debilitating condition of unknown cause. People who suffer from hyperhidrosis can sweat almost continuously from their foreheads, armpits, palms, and soles of the feet. Skin that is constantly moist can easily become chafed, macerated (softened and weakened), and infected; in addition, the copious sweat can lead to odor, social embarrassment, and expensive dry-cleaning bills. Until Botox, there was very little that could be done for this condition. Prescribed drugs had serious side effects, while antiperspirants provided little relief. Some sufferers went so far as to have their sweat glands removed or resorted to an operation called a sympathectomy, in which the sympathetic nerves to the affected area were cut. (The sympathetic nerves are part of the autonomic nervous system, which is not under our conscious control.)

Although sympathectomy has been effective for many people, it has several drawbacks. For one thing, it can prevent sweating in the entire upper body area, which can keep the body from cooling off when it needs to. For another, patients often develop a condition called *compensatory hyperhidrosis,* in which other parts of the body begin sweating excessively. Also, as with any surgical procedure, there is a risk of infection, and in 2 to 5 percent of patients sympathectomy doesn't work.

Enter Botox. Although at first it might seem strange that a toxin that prevents muscle movement could also prevent sweating, remember that Botox works by blocking nerve signals that tell a muscle to move. In the same way, it can block messages from the sympathetic nerves that tell sweat glands to produce perspiration. Doctors had noticed that when Botox was injected into the forehead for cosmetic reasons, sweating decreased.

Preventing hyperhidrosis has turned out to be one of the most successful medical uses of Botox. It almost always works and has few side effects. It works only on the areas that are injected, and as far as we know, no one has developed compensatory hyperhidrosis. At Institute Beauté we've been using Botox and Myobloc with excellent results for people with this condition.

In one case, we treated a law student who'd suffered her whole life with excessive perspiration of her hands and feet. She'd had a sympathectomy for her hands, which worked well. She didn't want to undergo surgery again, but her feet sweated so much that she was literally ruining her shoes. After one treatment with Botox, the perspiration on her feet subsided to a normal degree. Although she will probably need to repeat the treatments every six to fifteen months, the results to her seemed like a miracle. For us, it was simply another remarkable success story.

When used for weakening overactive muscles, Botox is injected into the muscle. For hyperhidrosis, Botox is injected into the skin of the area that produces excessive perspiration, avoiding the muscle. This is more painful and sometimes has a side effect of temporary and very slight weakness in the adjacent muscles.

For excessive sweating in the forehead, a number of very small, closely spaced injections of Botox are given throughout the area of greatest perspiration. In the armpit area, the doctor will first perform a test to determine the areas of greatest perspiration, then inject small amounts of Botox throughout those areas. For most patients, no anesthetic is necessary beyond a skin-numbing cream.

Although Botox treatments significantly reduce or even eliminate the most copious armpit sweating from the eccrine sweat glands, they have no effect on the other type of sweat glands, the apocrine glands, which produce "nervous" sweat. As a result, armpit odor may still be a problem, but it can be more easily controlled through cleanliness and deodorants.

Because they have so many nerves, we use a regional anesthetic (a nerve block) when treating the palms of the hands or soles of the feet. Once the area is numb, we inject the toxin in very small, precise doses along a grid covering the palm or sole of the foot (see illustration).

After being treated with Botox for hyperhidrosis, you will need to return for evaluation; in some cases you'll need a few supplemental injections to cover any small areas that are still producing excessive perspiration.

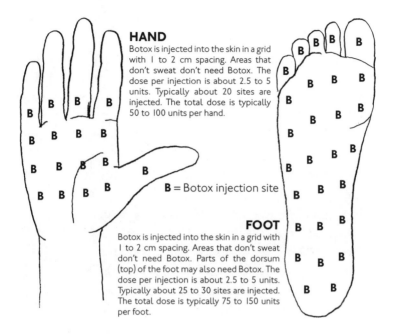

HAND
Botox is injected into the skin in a grid with 1 to 2 cm spacing. Areas that don't sweat don't need Botox. The dose per injection is about 2.5 to 5 units. Typically about 20 sites are injected. The total dose is typically 50 to 100 units per hand.

B = Botox injection site

FOOT
Botox is injected into the skin in a grid with 1 to 2 cm spacing. Areas that don't sweat don't need Botox. Parts of the dorsum (top) of the foot may also need Botox. The dose per injection is about 2.5 to 5 units. Typically about 25 to 30 sites are injected. The total dose is typically 75 to 150 units per foot.

Botox for hyperhidrosis lasts considerably longer than for many other purposes; in one study the effect lasted more than ten months in half the patients.

Jaw Disorders

Do you grind your teeth in your sleep? If so, you may be among the more than ten percent of the population who suffer from various spasmodic conditions of the jaw. These conditions are more than an annoyance—they can cause dental problems, ranging from worn to misaligned teeth, and in the case of teeth grinding, they may interfere with sleep. Although treatment studies are still in the preliminary stage, researchers have found that injections with Botox can alleviate these conditions in many cases.

Temporomandibular Joint Disorder (TMJ)

A quite common jaw problem, temporomandibular joint disorder (TMJ), is a malfunction of the jaw that results in jaw pain, headache, a "popping" noise, difficulty in opening or closing the mouth, and sometimes referred pain in the face, ear, shoulder, and neck. Standard treatment includes mouth appliances, physical therapy, and muscle relaxants. Since the cause is often misaligned teeth, orthodontia sometimes helps the condition.

In ongoing studies, researchers are now investigating the use of Botox to relax the jaw and ease the symptoms of TMJ. Although it's not yet a standard treatment, preliminary results indicate it is often effective in reducing the pain and discomfort associated with the condition. Canadian doctors Brian Freund and Marvin Schwartz report that in a recent study Botox produced a significant improvement in all major TMJ symptoms. For more information, check out their web site listed in Appendix A.

Migraine and Other Headaches

Botox is increasingly being used to treat migraine and tension-type headaches. It was first used for this purpose when doctors noticed that patients who were receiving Botox in their forehead reported fewer headaches.

Migraine is a particularly difficult condition to treat with standard medications. People with chronic migraines can be literally incapacitated when a headache strikes. Whereas a number of drugs and other therapies work for many patients, they are ineffective for others.

A number of studies have shown that Botox is effective in treating chronic headaches caused by muscle tension in the head or face muscles because it relaxes the involved muscles. The causes of migraine are still unknown, however, although many researchers suspect an oversensitive nervous system that responds to triggers, such as changes in the weather, particular foods, or changes in the body (such as monthly hormonal fluctuations in women).

Several fairly recent studies have examined the use of Botox in eliminating migraine headaches and have concluded that Botox works extremely well as a preventive. Researchers speculated that by relaxing the muscles of the head, Botox prevented muscle spasms from triggering or contributing to the severity of headaches. Treatment with Botox completely stopped migraines for some patients, and in most of the others it significantly reduced the frequency and severity of headaches.

If you are thinking of asking your doctor for Botox for your own headaches, you should be aware that most insurance companies will not cover its use for this purpose. This may change, however, as the use becomes more widespread and its effectiveness more apparent.

Spasticity in Adults Who Have Had Strokes

Spasticity, or muscle tightness, is often a consequence of strokes or other forms of brain damage. Those affected literally cannot relax their muscles, and the condition can be quite painful. Luckily, injections with Botox nearly always work with this condition, especially in the arm and leg muscles. Injections generally need to be repeated periodically.

Warts

Warts are considered a childhood affliction, but plenty of adults develop warts as well, usually on the feet and toes. These warts can become painful, especially if they are located on foot pressure points. Traditional therapy has focused on removing the warts (through cutting, freezing, or burning) and keeping the feet as dry as possible.

Those who suffer from warts can be miserable, because nothing they try seems to work. Even when the warts are removed, they tend to return, because the patients' feet still provide a warm, moist environment. Now we can use Botox to stop the feet from sweating and help patients get rid of warts once and for all. One man, a thirty-six-year-old lawyer, had suffered all his life from recurrent warts between his toes. He had surgical removal, which spread the warts, and he told us he had given up on ever finding relief. We injected Botox in the skin of his toes and the warts became a problem of the past. Botox created a less favorable environment for existing warts and halted the development of new warts. See the section on hyperhidrosis for more details on Botox injections for warts.

Other Conditions Under Study

The list of actual and possible medical uses for Botox is growing. The following conditions are currently being studied:

- **Chin muscle disorders:** The mentalis muscle is the main chin muscle. It's the muscle you use to pout (in conjunction with your lip muscles); it is also responsible for the quivering chin sometimes seen when people cry. When any condition occurs that causes the mentalis muscle to malfunction, such as the side effects of certain types of oral surgery, the result can be unsightly creasing and dimpling of the lower lip. Until recently, nothing much could be done about this condition, but it can now be easily fixed with Botox, with injections required every three or four months.

• **Facial tics:** There are many causes for facial tics, which are small, involuntary twitches of the facial muscles. There was no effective treatment for this embarrassing condition before Botox. By relaxing the affected facial muscles, Botox has proved help-ful in alleviating tics.

• **Myofascial pain** (severe muscle pain of unknown causes): This condition, characterized by extreme muscle pain usually in the neck and/or shoulders, is considered exceptionally difficult to treat. Most treatments, such as physical therapy and muscle relaxants, have had only limited success. A recent trial found that Botox reduced or eliminated the pain in a majority of participants, but there were a number of side effects, including flu-like symp-toms and muscle pain in other parts of the body. Ongoing tests will determine if Botox is a useful treatment for this condition.

• **Parkinson's disease:** Ongoing research indicates that Botox can be useful in treating many of the most troubling symptoms of Parkinson's disease.

• **Spastic bladder:** A spastic bladder is usually the result of spinal cord injury or a neurological dis-ease, such as multiple sclerosis. The patient may suffer from incontinence and urinary tract infec-tions because the bladder doesn't empty com-pletely. Preliminary studies have found that injecting Botox into the urethral sphincter can help to control this problem.

- **Stiff person syndrome:** In this odd and very rare condition of unknown cause the person gradually becomes very stiff, with muscle pain and sometimes excessive sweating. Stiff person syndrome has previously been treated with large doses of muscle relaxants, which can result in lethargy and drowsiness. Researchers have found that Botox can relax the muscles and relieve pain without side effects.

- **Stuttering:** The inability to speak fluently without inserting a number of extra syllables causes great social embarrassment for those who suffer from it. Stuttering is believed to be caused in part by over-stimulated vocal cords. Because Botox has been helpful in relieving spasms of the vocal cords, it has been tried as a treatment for stuttering. In ongoing trials the results have so far been mixed, but new techniques are being developed.

- **Tremors:** A number of conditions can cause tremors—continual shaking—of various parts of the body. Current research is using Botox to ease this condition. So far the toxin has produced promising results for head tremors, though tremors of the arms and legs respond less well.

Chapter 5
Botox and Beauty

It is in aesthetic procedures—rejuvenating the aging face and neck—that Botox seems most like a miracle drug. After all, what could be better than a treatment that works almost instantaneously, causes virtually no pain or side effects, and takes ten to fifteen years off your age?

How the Doctor Prepares It

Botox is prepared in the pharmaceutical laboratory for medical use by purifying and freeze-drying (lyophilization). It is then shipped on dry ice to doctors, who can store it in the freezer for more than a year. Your doctor prepares it fresh for use by mixing the freeze-dried material with preservative-free sterile saline solution. For maximum effectiveness, Botox must be used as fresh as possible, within twenty-four hours after it has been mixed with saline. Botox will retain activity for days in the refrigerator and might even work well, but its potency and effectiveness will be less certain.

What a Treatment Is Like

For any Botox procedure, your doctor might have you apply ice to the area a few minutes *before* treatment. This accomplishes two purposes: it causes the vessels in the skin to constrict (that is why your skin blanches), which will probably reduce the chance of bruising, and it helps decrease the minimal amount of pain associated with multiple injections. Ice can be valuable for the same reasons after the treatment with Botox.

When it's time for your treatment, you'll be seated upright in a medical chair. Your doctor will ask you to contract the muscle in the area being treated so that he or she can better target the injection into the muscle. Thus, if you're receiving injections for furrows between the eyes, you will be asked to frown. For some procedures, the doctor may use an electromyelogram—a device that helps your doctor locate the area of the muscle's greatest contraction. Using this device helps ensure that you will receive the right amount of toxin in the right place.

Depending on the area being treated, the average number of injections per muscle is three. With each injection you will feel a needle prick from the tiny microneedle, then a mild stinging or burning for a few seconds as the toxin is injected. Again depending on the area being treated, you may be asked to gently press a gauze pad against the injection site and/or hold ice to it for a few minutes.

The whole process takes from about ten minutes to half an hour, depending on the number of areas being treated. As soon as the series of injections is completed, you can go back to your regular activities.

Your doctor will probably ask you to refrain from bending over or lying down for approximately four hours after the injections until the toxin has had time to attach to the nerve–muscle connection. You will also be asked not to rub the area in order to prevent the toxin from spreading to adjacent muscles. For more information, see details on specific procedures in the next chapter.

What to Do Beforehand

We believe that the best outcomes result from good communication between doctors and patients. Thus, we encourage you to discuss any concerns you have with your doctor before the procedure. Let your physician known about all medical conditions and medications that might affect a successful outcome and recovery. In particular, we recommend letting your doctor know about any allergies you may have, including food and drug allergies, or allergies to environmental elements.

It's also important to give your doctor a list of all medications and supplements you are currently taking, including vitamins, herbs, and over-the-counter remedies. Some antiinflammatory medications, including aspirin, may lead to increased bruising from Botox injections. Vitamin E can also slightly increase the risk of bruising. Some antibiotics and other medicines can actually increase the potency of Botox, so your doctor may need to adjust the dosage.

During your initial meeting or just before your procedure, you will be asked to sign an informed consent release stating that you have been informed about all possible complications of Botox injections.

What to Do Afterwards

Your doctor will probably give you an ice pack to hold to the treated area for a few minutes after the procedure. This helps minimize bruising or postinjection discomfort and may help to keep the Botox localized in the injected areas. Botox usually takes two to four days or even a week to have its full effect. You might be asked to return after two weeks so that your doctor can evaluate the results of your treatment, although probably you won't need to see your doctor again until it's time for your next injections.

Remember that for maximum safety and effectiveness it's better to give too little toxin than too much, so it's possible that you won't receive the maximum desired effect after your treatment. If you feel the Botox hasn't worked sufficiently, if you notice asymmetry of the eyebrows or other areas, or if your eyebrow is drooping, phone your doctor and request a follow-up appointment at which you might receive a touch-up if the doctor deems it necessary. For some procedures, approximately 5 to 10 percent of patients might need a touch-up treatment. For more information, see details on specific procedures in the next chapter.

How Long It Lasts

Depending on the area being treated, one series of injections generally lasts three to six months, though in some cases the improved appearance can last up to a year. Although the studies are in the preliminary stages, Myobloc seems to last a slightly shorter time than Botox, but its effects are produced more quickly.

As the toxin wears off, your wrinkles will gradually return, but they won't be any worse than before the treatment. With repeated injections, the effects generally tend to last longer. There is some evidence that after prolonged treatment the affected muscles may become permanently weakened, so fewer treatments will be needed.

How Quickly the Effect Appears

You may notice some minor improvement within a day or two, but generally it takes three to seven days for the muscles to weaken. The cosmetic effect will continue to get better for several days to up to three weeks afterward. For most procedures you will see maximum results about five days after your Botox treatment. With Myobloc, the maximum effect appears somewhat sooner.

How Often It Needs to Be Injected

The amount of time between treatments varies considerably, depending on the person, the site of the injections, and how many treatments you have had in the past. Most procedures will need to be repeated within four to six months. Some, however, last considerably longer. See the sections on specific treatment sites in the next chapter for further details.

Possible Problems/Side Effects

Botox causes very few serious side effects. You may have small bruises or red marks at the sites of the injections that will fade in a few days. Occasionally people who have received forehead injections report a mild headache afterward, or, rarely, nausea. Some injections can cause mild muscle aches. It is also possible for an adjacent muscle to experience weakness, although this is usually temporary (one to three weeks) and minimal.

Rarely, the area around the injection will swell. If the swelling lasts more than a few hours, simple massage should help reduce it. (Caution: Do *not* massage the area in the hours immediately following your injection, since this could cause the toxin to spread to adjacent muscles.)

After you receive Botox, your doctor will probably ask you to refrain from bending over or from performing vigorous activities for several hours to prevent the toxin from migrating to an unwanted area. In rare cases, Botox injections around the eye area can cause your eyelid to droop, though this will wear off in two or three weeks. It is even rarer, but possible, for injections in the neck muscles (such as for stringy "turkey neck") to cause difficulty with swallowing. Be sure to discuss all these possibilities with your doctor before beginning treatment. For further details, see the individual sections on specific procedures in the next chapter.

Cost Guidelines

The cost of Botox treatments depends on your geographical location and where you go for treatment, as well as the areas you want treated. Usually, forehead injections are more expensive than those for crow's feet, because they require more of the toxin.

Some doctors charge by the injection, but most charge by the site. For example, the crow's feet on both sides, the forehead, and the glabella (between the eyes) are each considered separate sites and require a different number of injections. One well-known Beverly Hills plastic surgeon charges approximately $500 per site and says that an average patient will probably need to invest between $900 and $2,000 during the first year.

Depending on several factors, including the number of areas

treated and the geographic location of the doctor doing the treatment, you can probably count on a per-treatment range of $300 to $2,000. According to statistics published by the American Society of Aesthetic Plastic Surgery, the national average in 1999 was $432 per site. Costs were highest in the north-central and New England states and lowest in the south and west.

Be aware that with Botox, as with many valuable things in life, cheaper is not always better. What is your doctor's experience with Botox? Is the Botox fresh? Remember that the shelf life (refrigerator life) of Botox after it has been mixed with sterile saline is hours to a few days. Although it might still work quite well after five or more days, its strength probably decreases. (Myobloc has a refrigerator life of more than a year.) How much did the doctor dilute the Botox? Botox is expensive and there is a financial incentive to stretch it to the limit. If you get too small a dose, it may not work as well or for as long.

You probably already know that Botox injections are generally not covered by insurance for cosmetic purposes. However, many physicians make financing possible, as do some Internet sites (see Appendix A). As more people choose to rejuvenate their appearance through Botox, more sources of financing will undoubtedly become available.

Chapter 6
Rejuvenating the Upper Face

We are becoming so used to solving cosmetic problems with Botox that it's hard to believe it has only been used for this purpose for a little over a decade. In that time, thousands of doctors and hundreds of thousands of patients have experienced the seeming miracles that Botox can work on the upper face—relaxing wrinkles and getting rid of that tired, grumpy, or aged appearance.

In this chapter we take a closer look at the most common upper face cosmetic Botox procedures and what you can expect from each treatment.

Forehead Wrinkles

Those forehead lines that we think of as frown lines are among the first signs of aging. Depending on your skin type and environment, they can begin to appear as early as your twenties. Because they are caused primarily by facial expressions, they are also among the hardest wrinkles to treat. Even after a brow lift or surgical removal of the lines, they tend to return, simply because the forehead continues to move every time you smile, frown, or look surprised.

Numerous studies have shown that erasing forehead lines is one of the most successful uses of Botox. By eliminating excessive facial movements, Botox not only reduces or eliminates frown lines, it prevents them from recurring typically for three to six months.

What to Do Beforehand

There are no special precautions to take before Botox treatment. However, it's extremely important for you to communicate with your doctor about your expectations and concerns, and to let him or her know about any medications or supplements you are taking. For further details, see chapter 5.

The Procedure

The injections of Botox are made through a tiny needle, and the pain, if any, is minimal and short-lasting, so pain management is not necessary. Nevertheless, some doctors might have you apply ice to your face a few minutes before the procedure. You will be seated upright in a chair, then your doctor will ask you to raise your eyebrows strongly so that he or she can determine where to place the injections.

The number of injections will vary, depending on the number and severity of your forehead lines. You will probably be given between five and ten microinjections of Botox. These are usually placed in two rows at the top of the forehead and one or two short rows on either side of the face an inch or two above the eyebrows (see illustration).

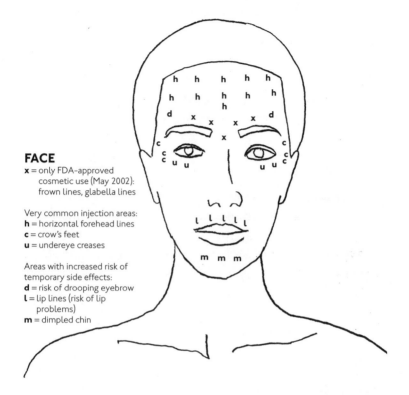

FACE

x = only FDA-approved cosmetic use (May 2002): frown lines, glabella lines

Very common injection areas:
h = horizontal forehead lines
c = crow's feet
u = undereye creases

Areas with increased risk of temporary side effects:
d = risk of drooping eyebrow
l = lip lines (risk of lip problems)
m = dimpled chin

A rule of thumb that the doctor follows is not to inject Botox closer than about 1.5 centimeters (a little over half an inch) above the outer eyebrow. This is to lessen the possibility of a droopy eyelid (ptosis).

What to Do Afterward

As with nearly all Botox facial procedures, you can resume your normal life immediately after the treatment—go back to work, go home, go shopping. However, your doctor will probably caution you not to bend over or perform strenuous exercises for the rest of the day. This precaution will help ensure that the Botox remains where it was injected and affects only the targeted muscles. You will also be asked not to rub the area, again to keep the toxin from spreading to adjacent tissues.

You might be asked to return to the doctor's office in two weeks to evaluate the success of the procedure. If you and your doctor agree that you need further treatment, you will receive another, more limited, series of Botox injections at that time.

How Quickly the Effect Appears

You may notice some minor improvement within a day or two, but generally it takes three to seven days for the muscles to weaken. The cosmetic effect will continue to get better for several days to up to three weeks afterward. For forehead lines, you should see maximum results three to five days after your Botox treatment.

How Often It Needs to Be Redone

For forehead wrinkles, one series of injections generally lasts three to six months. As the toxin wears off, your wrinkles will gradually return, but they won't be any worse than before the treatment. With repeated injections, the effects tend to last longer. There is some evidence that after prolonged treatment the affected muscles may become permanently weakened.

Possible Problems/Side Effects

The muscles that pull the forehead downward are stronger than those that pull it upward, so we inject both sets of muscles in a balanced way, to avoid brow droop. Special care must be taken in injecting men with very heavy brows, because if the muscles supporting the brow are weakened too much, the eyebrows can sag, making the upper eyelids appear baggy.

Some patients experience a feeling of heaviness in the forehead because of the sudden lack of muscle tone. This generally goes away after a few hours. Very rarely, the Botox can spread to adjacent muscles, causing the eyebrow or eyelid to droop. This problem goes away gradually as the Botox wears off, in a few weeks, or, rarely, in a few months.

Costs

Unless your doctor charges uniformly by the site, the cost for forehead lines will depend on the number and severity of your wrinkles. See the cost guidelines in chapter 5, and be sure to discuss this matter with your doctor.

Asymmetrical or Droopy Eyebrows

Writing in *Management of Facial Lines and Wrinkles,* Botox experts Drs. Jean and Alan Carruthers note that 80 percent of middle-aged women have eyebrows of noticeably different heights (the difference is usually one or two centimeters, or approximately one-third to three-quarters of an inch). This is because over time the muscles on one side of the face have become stronger than on the other, and the stronger muscles pull the eyebrow on their side down farther.

Amazingly, most women don't even realize they have an eyebrow discrepancy until it is pointed out to them. Luckily, uneven eyebrows can be corrected easily, either as a pretreatment for another procedure or as a stand-alone treatment, by injecting Botox into the muscles above the eyebrow on the side with the higher eyebrow, or below the side with the lower eyebrow. For those whose brows have begun to sag with middle age, Botox injections on both sides below the eyebrows will weaken the muscles that pull the brows down, elevating the brows and creating a more wide-awake, brighter look.

What to Do Beforehand

There are no special precautions to take beforehand. However, it's extremely important for you to communicate your expectations and concerns to your doctor. Tell your physician about medications or supplements you are taking. See chapter 5 for more information.

The Procedure

The injections of Botox are made through a tiny needle and the pain, if any, is minimal and short-lasting, so pain management is not necessary. Your doctor may have you apply ice to the area beforehand. As with other Botox facial procedures, you will be seated upright in a chair. Your doctor will ask you to strongly lower your eyebrows, then will inject a tiny amount of Botox into the muscles on the outside and below your eyebrows, or in the muscle of just one eyebrow if you want to even your brows.

What to Do Afterward

As with nearly all Botox facial procedures, you can resume your normal life immediately after the treatment—go back to work, go home, go shopping. However, your doctor will probably caution you not to bend over or perform strenuous exercises for the rest of the day. This precaution will ensure that the Botox remains where it was injected and affects only the targeted muscle. You will also be asked not to rub the area, again to keep the toxin from spreading to adjacent tissues.

You may be asked to return to the doctor's office in two weeks to evaluate the success of the procedure. If you and your doctor agree that you need further treatment, you will receive another Botox injection at that time.

How Quickly the Effect Appears

You may notice some minor improvement within a day or two, but generally it takes three to seven days for the muscle to weaken. The cosmetic effect will continue to improve for several days afterward. For uneven or droopy eyebrows, you should see maximum results about three days after your Botox treatment.

How Often It Needs to Be Redone

For droopy or asymmetrical eyebrows, one injection generally lasts three to six months. As the toxin wears off, your eyebrows will gradually return to the original position, but they won't look any worse than before the treatment. With repeated injections, the effects tend to last longer. There is some evidence that after prolonged treatment the affected muscles may become permanently weakened.

Possible Problems/Side Effects

In any procedure in the upper face, especially near your eyes, there is always a remote possibility that one or both of your eyelids could droop. In the unlikely event that this should occur, the problem will disappear on its own after a few weeks or a few months at most.

Costs

Because few injections are needed to even the eyebrows, this is one of the most economical Botox procedures. See the cost guidelines in chapter 5, and be sure to discuss possible costs with your doctor.

Around the Eyes (Crow's Feet)

What to Do Beforehand

There are no special precautions to take before Botox is injected. However, it's extremely important for you to communicate your expectations and concerns to your doctor. Let him or her know about medications or supplements you are taking. For further details, see chapter 5.

The Procedure

The injections of Botox are made through a tiny needle, and the pain, if any, is minimal and short-lasting, so pain management is not necessary. Your doctor may have you apply ice to the area beforehand. You will be seated upright in a chair, then your doctor will ask you to smile strongly so that he or she can determine where to place the injections.

This area is slightly more likely to get black and blue after injection, because injections for crow's feet are more superficial (inserted just below the skin), and the skin is thinner in this location. Black and blue marks typically last three to five days. Sometimes arnica, a homeopathic agent that is available over the counter, can help the bruises clear up more quickly.

You will be given one or two (or possibly more) microinjections of Botox toxin, typically in three sites on the outside of each eye: inside the upper part of the crow's feet just below the outside edge of your eyebrow; inside the central part of the crow's feet beside the corner of your eye; and inside the bottom part of the crow's feet just below the outer edge of your eye (see the illustration on page 67). Your doctor will probably ask you to smile strongly and may use a marker to indicate the upper, median, and lower positions of crow's feet. Then he or she will inject tiny amounts of toxin into each of the three areas for each eye.

What to Do Afterward

As with nearly all Botox facial procedures, you can resume your normal life immediately after the treatment—go back to work, go home, go shopping. However, your doctor will probably caution you not to bend over or perform strenuous exercises for the rest of the day. This precaution will ensure that the Botox remains in the injected area and affects only the targeted muscles. You will also be asked not to rub the area, again to keep the toxin from spreading to adjacent tissues.

You will probably be asked to return to the doctor's office in two weeks to evaluate the success of the procedure. If you and your doctor agree that you need further treatment, you will receive another series of Botox injections at that time.

How Quickly the Effect Appears

You may notice some minor improvement within a day or two, but generally it takes three to seven days for the muscles to weaken. The cosmetic effect will continue to improve for several days afterward. For crow's feet, you will see maximum results about five days after your Botox treatment.

How Often It Needs to Be Redone

For crow's feet, one series of injections generally lasts three to six months. As the toxin wears off, your crow's feet will gradually return, but they won't be any worse than before the treatment. With repeated injections, the effects tend to last longer. There is some evidence that after prolonged treatment the affected muscles may become permanently weakened.

Possible Problems/Side Effects

The most likely side effect of Botox injections for crow's feet is mild bruising in the area of the injection. If it occurs, it should only last for a day or two and can be covered up with makeup.

In any procedure in the upper face, especially near your eyes, there is always a remote possibility that one or both of your eyelids could droop. In the unlikely event that this should occur, the problem will disappear on its own after a few weeks or a few months at most.

Costs

Because few injections are needed to relax crow's feet, this is one of the most economical Botox procedures. See the cost guidelines in chapter 5, and be sure to discuss possible costs with your doctor.

Nose (Bunny Lines)

These horizontal lines appear along the sides of the nose in some people when they smile. The effect is caused by overactivity of the underlying muscle on either side of the nose. In some, the same muscle causes the nostrils to flare as well.

What to Do Beforehand

There are no special precautions to take before Botox injections. However, it's extremely important for you to communicate your expectations and concerns to your doctor. Let him or her know about medications or supplements you are taking. For further details, see chapter 5.

The Procedure

The injections of Botox are made through a tiny needle, and the pain, if any, is minimal and short-lasting, so pain management is not necessary. Your doctor may ask you to apply ice to the area a few minutes before the procedure. You will be seated upright in a chair, then your doctor will ask you to smile strongly so that he or she can determine where to place the injections on either side of your nose.

What to Do Afterward

As with nearly all Botox facial procedures, you can resume your normal life immediately after the treatment—go back to work, go home, go shopping. However, your doctor will probably caution you not to bend over or perform strenuous exercises for the rest of the day. This precaution will ensure that the Botox remains where it was injected and affects only the targeted muscles. You will also be asked not to rub the area, again to keep the toxin from spreading to adjacent tissues.

You might be asked to return to the doctor's office in two weeks to evaluate the success of the procedure. If you and your doctor agree that you need further treatment, you will receive another series of Botox injections at that time.

How Quickly the Effect Appears

You may notice some minor improvement within a day or two, but generally it takes three to seven days for the muscles to weaken. The cosmetic effect will continue to improve for several days afterward. For bunny lines you will see maximum results about five days after your Botox treatment.

How Often It Needs to Be Redone

For bunny lines, one series of injections generally lasts three to six months. As the toxin wears off, the lines will gradually return, but they won't be any worse than before the treatment. With repeated injections, the effects tend to last longer. There is some evidence that after prolonged treatment, the affected muscles may become permanently weakened.

Possible Problems/Side Effects

In any procedure in the upper face, especially near your eyes, there is always a remote possibility that one or both of your eyelids could droop. In the unlikely event that this should occur, the problem will disappear on its own after a few weeks or a few months at most.

Costs

Because few injections are needed to eliminate bunny lines, this is one of the most economical Botox procedures. See the cost guidelines in chapter 5, and be sure to discuss possible costs with your doctor.

Glabella (Between the Eyebrows)

Nearly everyone develops vertical furrows in the glabellar region—the area above the nose and between the eyebrows—usually beginning in the thirties, but in some people as early as the twenties.

What to Do Beforehand

There are no special precautions to take before Botox injections. However, it's extremely important for you to communicate your expectations and concerns to your doctor. Let him or her know about medications or supplements you are taking. For further details, see chapter 5.

The Procedure

The Botox injections are made through a tiny needle, and the pain, if any, is minimal and short-lasting, so pain management is not necessary. Nevertheless, your doctor may ask you to apply ice to the area a few minutes before the procedure. You will be seated upright in a chair, then your doctor will ask you to frown strongly so that he or she can determine where to place the injections.

For the glabellar area, you will probably be given five microinjections of Botox toxin. Two each will be placed on either side of your brow furrow, and one will be placed in the strong muscle just above it (see the illustration on page 67).

What to Do Afterward

As with nearly all Botox facial procedures, you can resume your normal life immediately after the treatment—go back to work, go home, go shopping. However, your doctor will probably caution you not to bend over or perform strenuous exercises for the rest of the day. This precaution will ensure that the Botox remains where it was injected and affects only the targeted muscles. You will also be asked not to rub the area, again to keep the toxin from spreading to adjacent tissues.

You may be asked to return to the doctor's office in two weeks to evaluate the success of the procedure. If you and your doctor agree that you need further treatment, you will receive another series of Botox injections at that time.

How Quickly the Effect Appears

You may notice some minor improvement within a day or two, but generally it takes three to seven days for the muscles to weaken. The cosmetic effect will continue to improve from several days to up to three weeks afterward. For brow furrows you will see maximum results about five days after your Botox treatment.

How Often It Needs to Be Redone

For brow furrows, one series of injections generally lasts three to six months or even longer. One patient reported that her first injection was still effective after two years. As the toxin wears off, your brow furrows will gradually return, but they won't be any worse than before the treatment. With repeated injections, the effects tend to last longer. There is some evidence that after prolonged treatment the affected muscles may become permanently weakened.

Possible Problems/Side Effects

In any procedure in the upper face, especially near your eyes, there is always a remote possibility that one or both of your eyelids could droop. Although rare, this is the most common complication with injections for brow furrows, and it is caused by the unintentional spread of the toxin to your eyelid muscles. The drooping eyelid, which usually appears a few weeks after the injection, is usually hardly noticeable and should disappear by itself within a week or two. To guard against this complication, be very careful not to rub the area around the injection for several hours.

Costs

Because few injections are needed to relax brow furrows, this is one of the most economical Botox procedures. See the cost guidelines in chapter 5, and be sure to discuss possible costs with your doctor.

Below the Eyes

Wrinkles below the eyes, especially those that become more pronounced when smiling, are much more common in mature people. Crinkly skin often accompanies these wrinkles. Both of these conditions are a reflection of life experience. And since both are caused by muscle movement, they can be improved by use of Botox.

What to Do Beforehand

There are no special precautions to take before Botox injections. However, it's extremely important for you to communicate your expectations and concerns to your doctor. Let him or her know about medications or supplements you are taking. For further details, see chapter 5.

The Procedure

The injections of Botox are made through a tiny needle, and the pain, if any, is minimal and short-lasting, so pain management is not necessary. Your doctor may ask you to apply ice to the area a few minutes before the procedure. You will be seated upright in a chair, then your doctor will ask you to smile strongly so that he or she can determine where to place the injections.

Typically your doctor will give you one to three Botox microinjections in the skin at the top of your cheekbone, toward the outside of your eye area (see illustration on page 67). The skin below your eye is very thin and the Botox is injected extremely superficially in this area, so the risk of bruising is increased. Applying ice prior to and/or after the injections will help to minimize black and blue marks. Also, for any injection, but especially in this area, your doctor or doctor's assistant may press on the area gently with gauze for about a minute after the injection (or they may ask you to do this), to help minimize the chance of bruising.

What to Do Afterward

As with nearly all Botox facial procedures, you can resume your normal life immediately after the treatment—go back to work, go home, go shopping. However, your doctor will probably caution you not to bend over or perform strenuous exercises for the rest of the day. This precaution will ensure that the Botox remains where it was injected and affects only the targeted muscles. You will also be asked not to rub the area, again to keep the toxin from spreading to adjacent tissues.

You may be asked to return to the doctor's office in two weeks to evaluate the success of the procedure. If you and your doctor agree that you need further treatment, you will receive another series of Botox injections at that time.

How Quickly the Effect Appears

You may notice some minor improvement within a day or two, but generally it takes three to seven days for the muscles to weaken. The cosmetic effect will continue to get better for several days afterward. For lines and crinkles beneath the eyes, you will see maximum results about five days after your Botox treatment.

How Often It Needs to Be Redone

For lines below the eyes, one series of injections generally lasts three to six months. As the toxin wears off, your lined, crinkled look will gradually return, but it won't be any worse than before the treatment. With repeated injections, the effects tend to last longer. There is some evidence that after prolonged treatment the affected muscles may become permanently weakened.

Possible Problems/Side Effects

Because the skin below the eyes is so thin, you are more likely to experience bruising (black and blue marks) than with Botox injections in other facial areas. A second possible, though unlikely, side effect is called "show"—where the lower eyelid droops, allowing the white of the eye below the iris to be visible. This isn't a medical problem and it disappears within a few weeks.

Costs

Because few injections are needed to improve lines below the eyes, this is one of the most economical Botox procedures. See the cost guidelines in chapter 5, and be sure to discuss possible costs with your doctor.

Chapter 7
Rejuvenating the Lower Face and Neck

When we first began using Botox to improve facial appearance, we concentrated on the upper part of the face—the forehead, eyebrows, and around the eyes—because the wrinkles in these locations were so clearly related to overactivity of the muscles and the downside of relaxing those muscles was minimal.

Dr. Alan Matarasso, a New York plastic surgeon and clinical associate professor of plastic surgery at Einstein Medical School, is one of the pioneers in using Botox to treat cosmetic problems in the lower part of the face. These procedures are still done far less often than those to the upper face, but their use is growing as doctors and patients experience good results.

"The main difference in injecting these areas is that we use much smaller doses," Dr. Matarasso says. "Obviously you can't go for complete paralysis of the muscles in the lower face." After all, he points out, it doesn't make much difference if you are unable to frown completely, but if the muscles around the mouth are paralyzed, your mouth won't work correctly.

"It's important for patients to realize that their expectations must be different in the lower face area," Dr. Matarasso stresses. "We look for a softening of the problem, rather than its complete elimination."

At Institute Beauté we use Botox with extreme caution on the lower face and neck, usually supplementing its effects with other treatments (for details, see chapter 8). We use very low doses of Botox, so the effects, although certainly good, are much less dramatic than for procedures on the upper part of the face.

If you decide to seek Botox treatment for any part of your lower face, we advise you to make certain that your doctor is experienced in this use of the drug. Although none of the side effects are life-threatening, any dysfunction of the mouth can be annoying and embarrassing, to say the least. In this chapter we take a closer look at the Botox procedures currently available for the lower face and neck, and what you can expect of each treatment.

Nasolabial Folds (Lines Between the Nose and Mouth)

Nasolabial folds are very prominent and often deep creases that form from the outside of the nose to the edges of the lips. They are caused by natural, continual muscular movement of the mouth—chewing, laughing, smiling, and talking. As we age, the skin becomes lax and begins to fall down over the creases, accentuating their appearance.

Although other cosmetic treatments, such as injectable fillers, can have a more dramatic effect on these lines than Botox, Botox treatments will soften their appearance and are a useful adjunct treatment. For more information on other treatments, see chapter 8.

What to Do Beforehand

There are no special precautions to take before Botox injections. However, it's extremely important for you to communicate your expectations and concerns to your doctor. Let him or her know about medications or supplements you are taking. For further details, see chapter 5.

The Procedure

The injections of Botox are made through a tiny needle, and the pain, if any, is minimal and short-lasting, so pain management is not necessary. Nevertheless, some doctors might ask you to apply ice to your face a few minutes before the procedure. You will be seated upright in a chair, then your doctor will ask you to smile strongly so that he or she can determine where to place the injections.

For nasolabial folds, you will probably be given one to three microinjections of Botox toxin in each side of the upper third of the crease, near the nose.

What to Do Afterward

As with nearly all Botox facial procedures, you can resume your normal life immediately after the treatment—go back to work, go home, go shopping. However, your doctor will probably caution you not to bend over or perform strenuous exercises for the rest of the day. This precaution will ensure that the Botox remains where it was injected and affects only the targeted muscles. You will also be asked not to rub the area, again to keep the toxin from spreading to adjacent tissues.

You might be asked to return to the doctor's office in two

weeks to evaluate the success of the procedure. If you and your doctor agree that you need further treatment, you will receive another series of Botox injections at that time.

How Quickly the Effect Appears

You may notice some minor improvement within a day or two, but generally it takes three to seven days for the muscles to weaken. The cosmetic effect will continue to improve for several days afterward. For nasolabial folds, you should see maximum results about five days after your Botox treatment.

How Often It Needs to Be Redone

For nasolabial folds, one series of injections generally lasts three to six months. As the toxin wears off, your lines will gradually return, but they won't be any worse than before the treatment. With repeated injections, the effects tend to last longer. There is some evidence that after prolonged treatment the affected muscles may become permanently weakened.

Possible Problems/Side Effects

Although you'll receive injections in several areas, each injection will contain only a very small amount of Botox toxin, because it's critical to leave the basic function of the muscles around the mouth undisturbed. Depending on your age and the severity of your nasolabial folds, you may need supplemental treatments, such as surgery, laser resurfacing, or injectable fillers, to fully correct the problem. For further details, see chapter 8.

Possible side effects, though rare, include mouth dysfunctions such as the inability to smile or talk properly, and even drooling. These side effects wear off in a few weeks to a few months.

Costs

Treatment for nasolabial folds will require a varying number of injections. See the cost guidelines in chapter 5, and be sure to discuss possible costs with your doctor.

Upper Lip Lines (Lipstick Lines)

These tiny, unsightly lines, sometimes called "lipstick lines" because of the tendency for lipstick to bleed into them, are usually the result of years of smoking. They are not generally a problem for men, because men have thicker skin than women and don't tend to show small, fine lines. Before Botox, the only treatments for these lines were injectable fillers such as collagen and laser or chemical resurfacing, both of which can be painful. For further details, see chapter 8. Botox can't completely eliminate upper lip lines, but it is a quick and relatively painless treatment, producing a softening that makes the lines seem to disappear.

What to Do Beforehand

There are no special precautions to take before Botox injections. However, it's extremely important for you to communicate your expectations and concerns to your doctor. Let him or her know about medications or supplements you are taking. For further details, see chapter 5.

The Procedure

The injections of Botox are made through a tiny needle, and the pain, if any, is minimal and short-lasting, so pain management is not necessary. Nevertheless, some doctors might ask you to apply ice to your face a few minutes before the procedure. You will be seated upright in a chair, then your doctor will ask you to purse your lips so that he or she can determine where to place the injections.

For upper lip lines, you will probably be given three to five microinjections of Botox toxin above the upper lip, in the moustache area (see illustration on page 67).

What to Do Afterward

As with nearly all Botox facial procedures, you can resume your normal life immediately after the treatment—go back to work, go home, go shopping. However, your doctor will probably caution you not to bend over or perform strenuous exercises for the rest of the day. This precaution will ensure that the Botox remains in the injected area and affects only the targeted muscles. You will also be asked not to rub the area, again to keep the toxin from spreading to adjacent tissues.

You may be asked to return to the doctor's office in two weeks to evaluate the success of the procedure. If you and your doctor agree that you need further treatment, you will receive another series of Botox injections at that time.

How Quickly the Effect Appears

You may notice some minor improvement within a day or two, but generally it takes three to seven days for the muscles to weaken. The cosmetic effect will continue to improve for several days afterward. For upper lip lines, you should see maximum results about five days after your Botox treatment.

How Often It Needs to Be Redone

For upper lip lines, one series of injections generally lasts three to six months. As the toxin wears off, your lines will gradually return, but they won't be any worse than before the treatment. With repeated injections, the effects tend to last longer. There is some evidence that after prolonged treatment the affected muscles may become permanently weakened.

Possible Problems/Side Effects

Although you'll receive injections in several areas, each injection will contain only a very small amount of Botox toxin, because it's critical to leave the basic function of the muscles around the mouth undisturbed. Depending on your age and the severity of your upper lip lines, you may need supplemental treatments, such as surgery, laser resurfacing, or injectable fillers, to fully correct the problem. For more information, see chapter 8.

Possible side effects, though rare, include mouth dysfunctions such as the inability to smile or talk properly, and even drooling. These side effects wear off in a few weeks to a few months.

Costs

Treatment for upper lip lines will require a varying number of injections; see the cost guidelines in chapter 5, and be sure to discuss possible costs with your doctor.

Marionette Lines (Creases from the Corners of the Mouth to the Chin)

"Marionette lines" are the often deep and prominent creases that form in middle age from the corners of the mouth to either side of the chin. They get their name from the hinged appearance they give to the lower third of the face, much like the face of a ventriloquist's puppet. Essentially, these creases are extensions of the nasiolabial folds, and, like the folds, are exacerbated by loose skin, which deepens their appearance.

Although other cosmetic treatments, such as injectable fillers, can have a more dramatic effect on these lines than Botox, Botox treatments will soften their appearance and are a useful adjunct treatment. For more information on other treatments, see chapter 8.

What to Do Beforehand

There are no special precautions to take before Botox injections. However, it's extremely important for you to communicate your expectations and concerns to your doctor. Let him or her know about medications or supplements you are taking. For further details, see chapter 5.

The Procedure

The injections of Botox are made through a tiny needle and the pain, if any, is minimal and short-lasting, so pain management is not necessary. Your doctor may ask you to hold ice to your face a few minutes before the procedure. You will be seated upright in a chair, then your doctor will ask you to smile strongly so that he or she can determine where to place the injections.

For marionette lines, you will be given one or more micro-injections of Botox toxin within each line. The number of injections and their exact placement will depend on how deep the lines are.

What to Do Afterward

As with nearly all Botox facial procedures, you can resume your normal life immediately after the treatment—go back to work, go home, go shopping. However, your doctor will probably caution you not to bend over or perform strenuous exercises for the rest of the day. This precaution will ensure that the Botox remains where it was injected and affects only the targeted muscles. You will also be asked not to rub the area, again to keep the toxin from spreading to adjacent tissues.

You might be asked to return to the doctor's office in two weeks to evaluate the success of the procedure. If you and your doctor agree that you need further treatment, you will receive another series of Botox injections at that time.

How Quickly the Effect Appears

You may notice some minor improvement within a day or two, but generally it takes three to seven days for the muscles to weaken. The cosmetic effect will continue to improve for several days afterward. For marionette lines, you should see maximum results about five days after your Botox treatment.

How Often It Needs to Be Redone

For marionette lines, one series of injections generally lasts three to six months. As the toxin wears off, your lines will gradually return, but they won't be any worse than before the treatment.

With repeated injections, the effects tend to last longer. There is some evidence that after prolonged treatment the affected muscles may become permanently weakened.

Possible Problems/Side Effects

Although you'll receive injections in several areas, each injection will contain only a very small amount of Botox toxin, because it's critical to leave the basic function of the muscles around the mouth undisturbed. Depending on your age and the severity of your marionette lines, you may need supplemental treatments, such as surgery, laser resurfacing, or injectable fillers, to fully correct the problem. For more information, see chapter 8.

Possible side effects, though rare, include mouth dysfunctions such as the inability to smile or talk properly, and even drooling. These side effects wear off in a few weeks to a few months.

Costs

Because treatment of marionette lines may require more injections than some other procedures, it may be among the more costly Botox procedures. See the cost guidelines in chapter 5, and be sure to discuss possible costs with your doctor.

Chin Wrinkles

As some people age, their mentalis muscle, the main muscle of the chin, begins to pull unevenly on the skin, causing wrinkles, small bumps or crinkles, and dimples to appear. There was little that could be done about this condition before Botox. Because of the possibility of side effects involving the mouth, only a very minimal dose is used, and the idea is to soften, rather than totally eliminate, the wrinkles and crinkles.

What to Do Beforehand

There are no special precautions to take before Botox injections. However, it's extremely important for you to communicate your expectations and concerns to your doctor. Let him or her know about medications or supplements you are taking. For further details, see chapter 5.

The Procedure

The injections of Botox are made through a tiny needle, and the pain, if any, is minimal and short-lasting, so pain management is not necessary. Nevertheless, some doctors might apply anesthetic cream to your face a few minutes before the procedure. You will be seated upright in a chair, then your doctor will ask you to strongly purse your lips so that he or she can determine where to place the injections.

For chin wrinkles, you will probably be given three to five microinjections of Botox toxin to either side of the chin (see illustration on page 67).

What to Do Afterward

As with nearly all Botox facial procedures, you can resume your normal life immediately after the treatment—go back to work, go home, go shopping. However, your doctor will probably caution you not to bend over or perform strenuous exercises for the rest of the day. This precaution will ensure that the Botox remains where it was injected and affects only the targeted muscles. You will also be asked not to rub the area, again to keep the toxin from spreading to adjacent tissues.

You might be asked to return to the doctor's office in two

weeks to evaluate the success of the procedure. If you and your doctor agree that you need further treatment, you will receive another series of Botox injections at that time.

How Quickly the Effect Appears

You may notice some minor improvement within a day or two, but generally it takes three to seven days for the muscles to weaken. The cosmetic effect will continue to improve for several days afterward. For chin wrinkles, you should see maximum results about three days after your Botox treatment.

How Often It Needs to Be Redone

For chin wrinkles, one series of injections generally lasts three to six months. As the toxin wears off, your wrinkles will gradually return, but they won't be any worse than before the treatment. With repeated injections, the effects tend to last longer. There is some evidence that after prolonged treatment the affected muscles may become permanently weakened.

Possible Problems/Side Effects

Although you'll receive injections in several areas, each injection will contain only a very small amount of Botox toxin, because it's critical to leave the basic function of the muscles in this area undisturbed. Depending on your age and the severity of your chin wrinkling, you may need supplemental treatments, such as surgery, laser resurfacing, or injectable fillers, to fully correct the problem. See chapter 8 for more information.

Possible side effects, though rare, include mouth dysfunctions such as the inability to smile or talk properly, and even drooling. These side effects wear off in a few weeks to a few months.

Costs

Because few injections are needed to alleviate chin wrinkles, this is one of the most economical Botox procedures. See the cost guidelines in chapter 5, and be sure to discuss possible costs with your doctor.

Neck Lines (Horizontal Neck Wrinkles)

Long before a person's neck becomes stringy and gaunt-looking (see "Turkey Neck"), horizontal wrinkles begin to form around the neck, like necklaces that proclaim aging. Before Botox, there was little that could be done for this condition short of plastic surgery.

Although we use Botox with care here, as with any procedure on the lower face, it is one of the most satisfying treatments, because the results are very good on nearly everyone.

What to Do Beforehand

You needn't take any special precautions or follow special instructions before having your neck treated with Botox, but your doctor will need to see you beforehand to discuss the probable outcome with you. Also, you should be aware of exactly what costs are involved.

Because the treatment takes so little time, removal of horizontal neck lines, like most Botox procedures, can be done as a "lunchtime" treatment.

The Procedure

The injections of Botox are made through a tiny needle and the pain, if any, is minimal and short-lasting, so pain management is not necessary. Your doctor might ask you to hold ice to your neck a few minutes before the procedure. (The ice helps to reduce bruising and discomfort.) When the doctor is ready to begin, you will be seated in an upright position while the skin of your neck is thoroughly cleaned with an alcohol swab and then allowed to dry. The alcohol must be completely evaporated or it might inactivate the Botox. Next, your doctor will ask you to contract your neck muscle by grimacing strongly. He or she will then use a microneedle to inject three to five doses of Botox into the muscles of the neck on either side. (The injected muscles, the platysma muscles, lie very close to the surface; for more information on them, see the section on "Turkey Neck" below.) The entire procedure should take only a few minutes.

What to Do Afterward

After receiving Botox injections, you will be asked not to bend over or perform strenuous exercises for the rest of the day. This precaution will ensure that the Botox remains where it was injected and affects only the targeted muscles. You will also be asked not to rub the area, again to keep the toxin from spreading to adjacent tissues.

You may be asked to return to the doctor's office in two weeks to evaluate the success of the procedure. If you and your doctor agree that you need further treatment, you will receive another series of Botox injections at that time.

How Quickly the Effect Appears

The muscles just beneath the skin of the neck will begin to weaken immediately after the injections, though it will probably take three to five days for you to see the improvement. The beneficial effects will increase over the next several weeks. It will take four to six months for these benefits to gradually disappear.

How Often It Needs to Be Redone

As the toxin loses effectiveness, your horizontal neck lines will begin to reappear. You will probably need a new treatment anywhere from four to eight months after the first.

Possible Problems/Side Effects

If the procedure is done by a qualified, experienced doctor, there are very few complications or side effects. Some possible reactions are slight bruising at the site of the injections and soreness or discomfort of the neck muscles.

You should be aware that there have also been reports of more serious complications involving hoarseness or the inability to swallow, but only in patients who have been treated with much larger doses of Botox for neck spasms. This is one reason it's so important to choose a fully qualified practitioner with experience in this cosmetic procedure.

Costs

The amount of Botox required will vary depending on the severity of your neck lines. See the cost guidelines in chapter 5, and be sure to discuss possible costs with your doctor.

Turkey Neck

Perhaps no other sign of aging is as discouraging as "turkey neck." Even if you have youthful-looking skin, hair, and teeth, the gaunt, stringy appearance of an aging neck can spoil the illusion. Before the use of Botox, there was nothing to do except cover it up—with a scarf or turtleneck—or resort to plastic surgery, which can require a complicated series of procedures involving the neck and lower facial muscles.

Not only are these surgical procedures costly, but they take three weeks or more of downtime for healing. They also carry the risk of side effects, including pain or discomfort when you move your neck, injury to the parotid (salivary) glands, and injury to the facial nerves.

Although Botox injections for an aging neck are less well studied than some of the other cosmetic uses, a growing number of doctors have been using this treatment on their patients with excellent results. At Institute Beauté, we've used it for several years, usually in conjunction with other procedures. We've never had a problem with side effects, and our patients have mostly been thrilled with the results.

To understand how Botox helps an aging neck, let's take a closer look at the muscles of the neck and how they affect the appearance of the neck and lower face. The muscle that causes all the trouble is a wide, flat, frontal neck muscle that lies directly beneath the skin, the platysma. Also known as the neck muscle of facial expression, the platysma's main function is to lower your lower lip and drop your jaw. It also helps tighten the skin over your neck. To see the platysma at work, tense your neck muscles and drop your jaw.

With age, the platysma loses tone and begins to separate into bands, which form those ugly strings in the aging neck. Without support in the center, your neck begins to angle downward, producing a "turkey gobbler" appearance. At the same time, the platysma can pull on the bottom part of your face, accentuating jowls on the lower part of your jawline. Other factors affecting the appearance of the neck include fatty deposits under the chin, which are common after middle age, and sun damage, causing spotted, inelastic skin, neither of which Botox can help directly.

Before deciding if you are a good candidate for Botox, your

physician will need to make a careful assessment of your particular anatomy. This is because the platysma muscles are attached in various ways.

The three ways the muscles can attach are type I, the most common (approximately 75 percent of all people), in which the platysma muscles on either side meet just below the chin; type II, in which the muscles on either side meet somewhat lower on the neck, forming one continuous band (15 percent of all people); and type III, in which the muscle fibers on each side don't meet their counterparts (10 percent of all people).

For types I and II, Botox injections can generally have a positive, rejuvenating effect on the neck, in some cases returning it to an unlined, youthful appearance. However, people with type III necks may also need to have liposuction of the underlying fat pads for a satisfactory outcome.

There is some evidence that starting Botox treatments for the neck at an early age may help prevent some of the changes that lead to turkey neck and other unattractive changes. But no matter what your age or the condition of your neck, Botox injections will probably improve its appearance.

According to Dr. Alan Matarasso, who conducted one of the studies on Botox for neck rejuvenation, Botox has a number of advantages as a treatment for the aging neck. "No preparation is required, the results are rapid, it is highly successful and predictable, it does not require systematic anesthesia, and patients experience little discomfort."

What to Do Beforehand

You needn't take any special precautions or follow special instructions before having your neck treated with Botox, but your doctor will need to see you beforehand to evaluate the position of your platysma muscles and the degree to which your neck is aging. At this time, the doctor will also discuss the probable outcome with you, as well as costs. Because the treatment takes so little time, neck rejuvenation, like most Botox procedures, can be done as a "lunchtime" treatment.

The Procedure

The injections of Botox are made through a tiny needle, and the pain, if any, is minimal and short-lasting, so pain management is not necessary. Your doctor might apply anesthetic cream or ice to your neck a few minutes before the procedure.

When the doctor is ready to begin, you will be seated in an upright position while the skin of your neck is thoroughly cleaned with an alcohol swab. The alcohol must be completely evaporated before the injections are given or it might inactivate the Botox. Next, your doctor will ask you to contract your platysma muscle by grimacing so that he or she can identify all of its bands.

While you continue to grimace, the doctor will grasp each individual muscle band, and, holding it firmly, use a microneedle to inject minute amounts of Botox into the muscle band from the jawline to the lower neck. The doctor will repeat injections with the other muscle bands. The entire procedure should take only a few minutes (see illustration on page 101).

The needles are extremely small and cause little pain. Some patients have likened the experience to a mild insect sting.

What to Do Afterward

After receiving Botox injections, you will be asked not to bend over or perform strenuous exercises for the rest of the day. This precaution will ensure that the Botox remains where it was injected and affects only the targeted muscles. You will also be asked not to rub the area, again to keep the toxin from spreading to adjacent tissues.

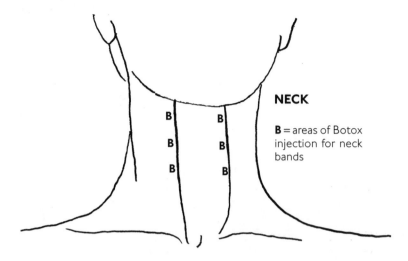

NECK

B = areas of Botox injection for neck bands

You may be asked to return to the doctor's office in two weeks to evaluate the success of the procedure. If you and your doctor agree that you need further treatment, you will receive another series of Botox injections at that time.

How Quickly the Effect Appears

The platysma muscle will begin to weaken immediately after the injections, though it will probably take three to five days for you to see an improvement in the appearance of your neck. The improvement will increase over the next several weeks, and the effects of the Botox will wear off gradually over four to six months.

Bear in mind that Botox can only help the muscles of the neck. If you have loose, wrinkly neck skin because of sun damage and/or age, the skin will not look much better after your treatment. For optimal neck appearance, you will require further treatment—a peel, CoolTouch laser treatments, injectable implants, or even plastic surgery. For details, see chapter 8.

How Often It Needs to Be Redone

As the toxin wears off, your neck bands will begin to reappear. You will probably need a new treatment from four to eight months after the first. Although this procedure for the neck is still relatively new, our experience is that the effects last longer with each treatment.

Possible Problems/Side Effects

If the Botox injections are given by a qualified and experienced doctor, there are very few complications or side effects. Some possible reactions are slight bruising at the site of the injections (this is slightly more common than for some other Botox injections because the injections are very superficial) and soreness or discomfort of the neck muscles. Some patients have reported mild weakness of the neck when performing sit-ups for one or two weeks after the procedure.

There have also been reports of more serious complications involving hoarseness or the inability to swallow, but only in patients who have been treated with much larger doses of Botox for neck spasms. This is one reason it's so important to choose a fully qualified physician with experience in this cosmetic procedure. If the injections are not done correctly, the chances increase for more serious side effects.

Costs

Because neck rejuvenation involves multiple injections of several platysma bands and might require as much as an entire vial of Botox (100 units), it is more costly than some other Botox procedures. See the cost guidelines in chapter 5, and be sure to discuss possible costs with your doctor.

Chapter 8
When Botox
Is Not Enough

When it comes to looking younger, Botox is one of the greatest treatments around, because it's widely available, has minimal side effects, and provides near-instant results.

But even Botox can't do everything. For some people, especially those with profound aging changes, other treatments will be necessary in order for them to look their very best. Often, *combining* Botox with these procedures produces better results than using either treatment alone.

We believe that if you begin using Botox early enough, you may be able to put off more drastic treatments indefinitely, or maybe forever. But if you already have obvious signs of aging, or feel you need or want more serious treatments, here are the latest, most cutting-edge ways to improve and rejuvenate your looks.

The Main Rejuvenating Treatments

CoolTouch Laser

Many of the patients we treat at Institute Beauté feel that the CoolTouch laser produces magical results. One of a number of laser tools designed to enhance the skin's appearance, the CoolTouch laser targets the slightly deeper layers of your skin while a cooling spray protects the skin surface. Thus, CoolTouch actually rejuvenates your skin from the inside out, stimulating the formation of new collagen and even elastin, the structural materials that give skin its plumpness and resilience.

Each CoolTouch treatment lasts 15 or 20 minutes, with at least two to four treatments a minimum of three weeks apart recommended initially. While most people experience some very transient burning, especially on the upper lip, this is over in seconds. There is no recovery time, and the skin usually looks better right away. The results may be subtle at first, but they become dramatic as time passes and new collagen is produced, reaching a maximum result, at about six months after the last treatment, that should last for years.

As the skin begins to fill out, superficial wrinkles disappear along with that aging, gaunt look. CoolTouch can be used on any part of your body—even the bottoms of feet—to restore some of the natural collagen padding that has disappeared with age.

Injectable Implants

Miraculous space-age products still awaiting FDA approval, such as Artecoll, Reviderm, Restylane, Rofilan, Perlane, New Fill, and others, can be used to fill in deep lines and wrinkles, as well as acne scars. Unlike the old-fashioned collagen or fat injections, these new injectables are long-lasting and carry little risk of allergic reaction or rejection. When used in conjunction with Botox, they can create a smooth and youthful complexion in the areas that are quickest to show age and stress, such as the forehead and around the mouth.

Microdermabrasion

Microdermabrasion, which is one of our most popular procedures, offers the results of a peel without the downtime. Microdermabrasion employs a controlled fine mist of microscopic aluminum oxide (or sodium chloride) crystals that are sprayed on the top layers of skin, causing exfoliation; this dead skin is immediately vacuumed away, thereby gradually diminishing fine lines, wrinkles, acne scars, and discoloration. Microdermabrasion requires no anesthesia and only takes about thirty minutes, so it's often referred to as the "lunchtime" peel.

Aura Laser

The Aura is one of several lasers that target specific skin problems. Using an intense green light, the Aura targets brownish, reddish, or dark pigmentation, eliminating or softening the appearance of port wine stains, birth marks, age spots, spider veins, rosacea, and other pigmented areas. It affects the surface appearance of the skin only and doesn't help wrinkles, furrows, or fine lines.

Intense Pulsed Light (IPL)

This new nonsurgical treatment is said by its proponents to work wonders on aging skin. Instead of a laser, which applies an intense beam of a specific wavelength of light to the targeted part of the skin, IPL uses intense pulses of broad-spectrum light—light that contains many different wavelengths—to deliver heat energy to the skin or just beneath the skin. Often a colored filter is used to narrow the spectrum, which is still not the pure single color (single wavelength) of a laser.

Like CoolTouch laser treatments, IPL can stimulate formation of new collagen beneath the skin. It can also affect several more superficial aging signs, diminishing or erasing redness, spider veins (what some people call broken capillaries), fine lines, large pores, and acne scars. This procedure can improve an aging appearance on the entire face as well as the neck, chest, and backs of the hands. IPL can also be used for long-term removal of unwanted hair.

Laser and Chemical Resurfacing

These treatments, which we don't usually recommend, rejuvenate your skin by literally removing the surface layers. When the new skin grows back, it is generally blemish- and wrinkle-free, with a youthful resilience. The obvious disadvantages to these procedures include discomfort, lengthy downtime for healing, and a shiny, "boiled" look that can persist for months or years.

Another drawback to resurfacing is that in many patients the movement-associated wrinkles, such as those between and above the eyebrows, start to recur within six to twelve months.

Plastic Surgery

One of the oldest procedures in the book, plastic surgery, which can be performed on any part of the face, neck, or body, generally tightens loose muscles while eliminating excess, sagging skin. Among the many drawbacks are that it is, after all, surgery, with all its downtime and risks; the results are by no means guaranteed; and an unnatural or asymmetrical appearance is possible. However, only plastic surgery can correct some problems, including a very aged appearance or an extremely lined and baggy face and neck.

Some plastic surgery procedures target only a limited part of the face, such as a brow lift or blepharoplasty (eyelid surgery). Others involve a series of procedures done in concert, such as a complete face-lift or a neck-lift combined with liposuction.

Combining Botox with Other Treatments

We and other physicians increasingly find that Botox improves the outcome of other procedures, especially those involving areas where muscle movement is an important factor. For example, by relaxing muscles and evening out the face, Botox generally makes it easier for a plastic surgeon to offer more accurate treatment.

Botox is especially helpful as an adjunctive treatment to injectable implants for nasolabial folds and marionette lines. By weakening the muscle that causes the line or crease, Botox can help prevent the injectable implant from moving. Useful as they are, injectable implants are liquid and are subject to slight movement for hours to a few days after they are injected. This is good, in that they can then be gently molded into the best position and shape. But it's also a problem, because if you sleep with pressure on the implant before it has "fixed" in place, it might move or mold in an unwanted way. Muscle action can also slightly displace the implant, possibly even accentuating a line or a wrinkle. To avoid the former problem, sleep on your back. To avoid the latter, ask your doctor to combine the implant treatment with a Botox treatment, which weakens the muscles and reduces movement of the implant away from the crevice or line it was intended to fill.

Those who are having laser resurfacing of the upper part of the face will also have a much better result if they are pretreated with Botox. Using Botox to relax the muscles responsible for crow's feet, frown lines, and bunny lines can prevent the wrinkling from quickly returning to the newly resurfaced skin.

A new study also demonstrates that using Botox *after* resurfacing can improve the appearance of the new skin and prevent or delay recurrence of the unwanted wrinkles and furrows.

Botox is increasingly used before blepharoplasty (eyelid surgery). Pretreating the crow's feet extending from the corners of the eyelids not only improves the result after surgery but makes the scars less visible.

Dr. Alan Matarasso likes to use Botox as an adjunct to neck surgery. "It's good for getting the things surgery didn't correct," he reports.

In our own practice, we find Botox extremely useful both as a stand-alone treatment and in conjunction with other procedures. For example, although CoolTouch laser and injectable implants are great for minimizing deep and superficial wrinkles, they do nothing for the underlying problem of hyperactive muscles, which is, so to speak, Botox's specialty.

Just as rejuvenating products and tools are constantly being developed, so the value of Botox grows every day. If properly orchestrated in their use, Botox, CoolTouch laser (and other lasers), injectable implants, microdermabrasion, and other peels can work in concert to create a more fully harmonized, rejuvenated appearance—a more beautiful and youthful you.

When Botox Is Not Enough

Comparing Botox and Other Cosmetic Procedures

TREATMENT	DYNAMIC DEEP WRINKLES	FINE LINES	SAGGING SKIN	NECK BANDS	SPOTS AND BLEMISHES
Botox	Good results	Some help	Some help	Good results	No effect
Injectable implants	Good results	Some help	Fair results	Fair results	no effect
CoolTouch laser	Fair results	Good results	Fair results	Some help	No effect
Aura laser (green lasers)	No effect	Minimal results	No effect	No effect	Good to excellent results
Intense pulsed light (IPL)	No effect	Fair to good results	Minimal to fair results	Minimal results	Good results
Microdermabasion	No effect	Fair results	No effect	No effect	Good results
Plastic surgery	Fair to good results	Fair results	Good results	Good results	No effect
Deep peel	Fair to good results	Good results	Fair results	No effect	Good results

Chapter 9
How Botox
Enhances Other
Cosmetic Procedures

Now that Botox has been approved by the FDA for cosmetic use, and with all the media hype about Botox parties and the ease and reliability of Botox, we are becoming aware of a growing phenomenon of "Botox mills," or cosmetic treatment centers that may be staffed by less-than-fully-qualified medical professionals. Although you may be tempted to go to a discount Botox clinic, it's simply not worth saving a few dollars—or even a few hundred dollars—if an unsightly appearance is the result.

Never doubt that the best outcome is assured only by choosing an experienced physician who knows how much toxin to inject and precisely where to inject it. If too much Botox is injected, the result could be a bland and expressionless face; if too little is used, the wrinkles and crow's feet will remain. In addition, if the toxin is not injected in *precisely* the right position, neighboring muscles could be affected, resulting in a drooping eyelid or uneven results, such as one eyebrow being raised much higher than the other (called by a nurse who assists her physician husband in aesthetic treatments "the Mr. Spock Look").

The American Society for Aesthetic Plastic Surgery reports that Botox injections are being offered in some areas by untrained personnel in such non-medical environments as salons, gyms, hotel rooms, and even home offices. We can't stress enough how dangerous this can be. Not only are you risking a treatment with the wrong amount of Botox injected in the wrong place, but you're also risking infection from unsanitary conditions.

According to Dr. Malcolm Paul of the American Society for Aesthetic Plastic Surgery, "People may think that the procedure is only a simple injection and not realize that it requires an in-depth knowledge of the facial muscles and the relationship of these muscles to normal facial movement." This is why, Dr. Paul stresses, it's essential to choose a board-certified physician with appropriate training and experience.

Dr. Michael B. Stevens, a cosmetic plastic surgeon with practices in both Beverly Hills and Visalia, California, has a Ph.D. in anatomy, which helps him to tailor each treatment to the individual patient's needs. According to his web site, Dr. Stevens's experience and individualized approach minimize the need for touch-up treatments. An administrator for Dr. Stevens says that patients often drive long distances to be treated by Dr. Stevens because his results are better than some patients have received from other, less knowledgeable and experienced, practitioners.

Another important consideration is aesthetics. Not every doctor has an eye for beauty. Although he or she may be able to competently inject the correct amount of Botox, it's important to work with a doctor who can envision your entire face as it is now and as it will look after the treatments. One of our patients, Lorena, is a real Botox pioneer who began receiving injections twelve years ago, when she was only forty.

Lorena first started coming to Institute Beauté about three years ago, after a friend recommended us. Now, she says, she wouldn't go anywhere else. "What I like is that you have such a good eye," she told us. "With other doctors, I'd have to tell them where I needed the shots. With you, you always know, sometimes before I do."

How to Find a Doctor for Botox Treatments

Most doctors with experience in offering cosmetic Botox treatments are plastic surgeons and dermatologists. Many other doctors in other specialties also use Botox for medical purposes and may offer cosmetic treatments as well. No matter what your doctor's specialty, be certain that he or she has ample experience using Botox for the procedure you are contemplating. It's best to choose someone with experience in a wide variety of cosmetic techniques, because only someone with that background can determine if Botox is right for you, or if you would get better results from a different procedure, or by combining another procedure with Botox.

One of the best ways to find a good doctor is to ask around. Perhaps your family doctor can recommend someone. If you have friends who've had Botox, ask them to tell you about their experience and whether they would recommend their doctor. Other places to get tips are beauty parlors and health clubs. Botox has become so popular that nearly everyone knows someone who's had the injections.

Another good way to find a qualified doctor is to check out your local medical societies or use one of the many physician locator services on the Internet. See Appendix A, which lists a number of relevant web sites.

Questions to Ask Your Doctor

As we stressed in an earlier chapter, good communication between doctor and patient is the key to a successful outcome in Botox treatments or any other procedures. When you meet with your physician for the first time, don't hesitate to share your concerns. Although you may feel nervous asking the doctor about his or her credentials and experience, a reputable physician will readily supply this and other information that's directly relevant to your planned procedure.

The physician should also have a prepared sheet explaining what to expect after the procedure (pain, swelling, restrictions on activity, medications to take or avoid) or should give you detailed instructions on postprocedure care.

In addition to the obvious questions about costs and financing, you might ask to see before-and-after photos or videotapes of patients who have had the same procedure you are considering. Other questions you may want to ask include:

- **Are my desired results realistic? If not, what is the best outcome I can hope for?** Beware of doctors who "promise the moon." While nearly everyone will benefit from Botox injections, the degree of improvement in your appearance will depend on a number of factors, including your age, type of skin, degree of sun damage, and underlying muscular structure. If you currently look like Yoda, Botox alone can't make you into Barbie.

- **Is there another procedure that would give me a better result than Botox?** As we've stressed throughout this book, Botox can't do everything.

For many problems, such as old acne scars or severely sun-damaged skin, Botox is useless. Your physician should mention alternative treatments if they are more appropriate.

- **How many times have you performed this particular procedure with Botox? How long have you been doing this procedure?** If your doctor is fully qualified, he or she won't mind giving you a candid answer to these questions.

- **How many of your patients have had complications?** Again, a competent and qualified doctor will have no qualms about sharing this information.

- **Can I contact some of your previous patients?** Don't be afraid to ask to speak to other patients, and when you do, ask for their candid appraisal, both of the procedure and their interaction with the doctor.

- **If I'm not pleased with the outcome, will you repeat or correct the treatment without charging me extra?** Some doctors will ask you to return approximately two weeks after your treatment for a follow-up visit, at which time any additional injections can be done if needed. If the original results were unsatisfactory, a reputable doctor should be willing to touch up the treatment as necessary for no extra charge.

Cautions

While the majority of doctors are ethical and dedicated to their patients' welfare, there are bad apples in every bunch, including some who may try to make an extra profit out of Botox by using an overly diluted or stale preparation. Although the amount of saline mixed with Botox doesn't need to be exact down to the milliliter, the administered dosage does make a difference. If a doctor charges you much less than the going rate per injection or per site, it's possible that he or she is stretching the Botox by overdiluting it, or using Botox that isn't fresh. Beware of doctors who:

- Will not show you their certification
- Tell you that Botox will solve all of your cosmetic problems
- Refuse to let you speak to previous patients
- Charge much less than the going rate
- Are too rushed to give you adequate time for consultation before your procedure

How to Keep Your Great New Look

Botox is not a magic bullet. While it can certainly improve your appearance at any age, it cannot alone make up for years of neglect, nor can it keep you looking young without some effort on your part.

Plastic surgeon Dr. Alan Matarasso offers the following suggestions, with which we wholeheartedly agree. Beginning as soon as you possibly can, practice good health habits. Eat well and exercise, and above all:

- **Avoid smoking,** which compromises the blood supply to your face, producing premature wrinkling and a sallow complexion.

- **Watch your weight.** Or, more accurately and perhaps surprisingly, avoid extreme fluctuations in your weight. Constantly gaining and losing weight has a devastating effect on your skin, and the older you become, the worse the effects. By the time you are middle-aged, losing a few pounds will produce wrinkled, lax skin on your face and elsewhere on your body.

- **Use sun protection!** No matter where you live, always use at least a 30 SPF sunscreen when you go outside. Remember that sun damage is cumulative. Every little bit hurts. When you're going to be out during the prime sun hours of 10 A.M. to 3 P.M., wear long sleeves and a brimmed hat. The sooner in life you start, the better. Ninety percent of all sun damage occurs before age twenty-two.

Staying Young Longer

Nearly all the lines and wrinkles we've talked about in this book are dynamic wrinkles caused by muscle movement. One of the facts of life is that with time and aging these lines can become permanent in the skin, even when the muscles are not consciously being used. While Botox definitely can improve the appearance of these lines, they will still show, even when you are wearing a neutral expression.

However, it's possible that if you start early enough, those permanent changes in the skin will never occur, or if they do, they will be far less obvious. For your own best possible look over a lifetime, we urge you to practice early intervention. Don't wait until your wrinkle or line problem is hopeless—go for treatment when it first becomes noticeable, and it may not get much worse for a very long time.

Bear in mind that there is no one right age for beginning Botox treatments. Someone who has spent a great deal of time in the sun might need them at age twenty-six, whereas someone in her mid-thirties might not need to do anything for several more years.

Skin Products That Can Help

Finally, after you have received Botox treatments, practice all the good habits already listed, especially with regard to no smoking, avoiding weight fluctuations, and getting good sun protection. In addition, use one or more prescription skin products that have been proven to prevent and heal superficial aging changes. Among those we recommend are the following:

- **Renova:** This is the best-known of the prescription creams derived from Tretinoin, a natural substance that is similar to Vitamin A. It was developed originally to treat severe acne; early researchers noticed that in addition to zapping pimples, Retin-A made the skin smoother, clearer, and firmer. It actually works within the skin, rejuvenating it on the deeper levels. Renova was the first product approved by the FDA to treat sun-damaged skin.

- **Vitamin C serums and creams:** A number of prescription creams and lotions contain concentrated vitamin C (the L form of ascorbic acid is best), which is an anti–free radical antioxidant that has also been proven to stimulate the formation of new collagen and help reverse superficial aging changes. Some of these preparations also contain vitamin E, which possesses antioxidizing and moisturizing properties.

- **Kinerase (Furfuryladenine):** This new product is said by some to work as well as Renova. Derived from a growth factor in plants, Kinerase is designed to be applied to the neck, shoulders, chest, and hands. In addition to reducing the appearance of fine lines and wrinkles, Kinerase also acts as an extremely good moisturizer.

- **Alpha-hydroxy and glycolic acid creams and lotions:** These preparations hasten the removal of outer, drab, wrinkled layers of skin, producing a smoother, less blemished surface. While they don't affect your skin on the deeper levels, as the three previous products do, they can improve the appearance of your skin after Botox treatments.

AVOIDING BOTOX RESISTANCE

A very small number of patients don't respond to Botox at all. A larger group, from 3 to 10 percent, develop resistance after they have used it several times. The cause of Botox resistance isn't known, but it may have something to do with the way Botox is prepared. Since Myobloc isn't freeze-dried, it may be less likely to cause resistance in its users. To avoid Botox resistance, experts recommend that you:

• Receive treatments as infrequently as possible, no more than once every three months.

• Ask your doctor to use the lowest possible effective dose.

• Ask your doctor to slightly alter the site of injections, if possible.

• Switch to Myobloc if resistance develops.

Chapter 10
Questions

By now we hope you have learned all you hoped to know about Botox and how it can rejuvenate your appearance and help with a host of common health problems. Whether you decide to have your own wrinkles erased or that Botox is just not for you, we hope that what you have read in this book will help you take a proactive approach to the care of your skin. For the best-looking skin for you, whatever your age, remember to minimize your sun exposure, use sunscreen, and treat your skin to one or more of the rejuvenating preparations mentioned in chapter 9.

Following are some of the questions our patients most commonly ask us, along with a short answer and reference to a more thorough discussion earlier in the book.

Can I lose sensitivity or become allergic to Botox?

There are no known cases of anyone having an allergic reaction to Botox. However, approximately 3 to 10 percent of patients receiving Botox treatments eventually develop antibodies that cause them to stop responding to it. This is most likely for those receiving relatively large amounts of Botox for medical conditions, but it can also happen with cosmetic procedures.

Fortunately, those who have stopped responding to Botox can probably obtain equally good results from Myobloc, which is made from Botulinum B and has very similar, if not identical, effects. For more information on Myobloc, see chapter 3.

What results can I expect from Botox cosmetic treatments?

No one can promise that you will regain all of your lost youth and be ready to step onto the cover of *Vogue* after Botox injections, but statistics show that Botox patients are nearly 100 percent pleased with the results of their treatments.

Your doctor can help you form a realistic assessment of what to expect by taking a look at your age, your skin type, and to a certain extent, your lifestyle. (For example, skin of any age that has spent a great deal of time in the sun will be more damaged and respond less dramatically than skin that has been covered up and protected with sunscreen.)

In general, the younger you are, the better your results. For patients in their twenties and thirties who have relatively thin, smooth skin, Botox can virtually eliminate frown lines. Older patients, or those who have thicker, oily skin, will still have good results, but their wrinkles will be softened rather than eliminated.

The area being treated also makes a difference. Treatments to the upper part of the face (crow's feet, frown lines) generally produce a more dramatic improvement than treatments to the lower part (nasolabial folds, "marionette" lines). For more detailed answers, see information under the specific procedures in chapters 6 and 7.

Does Botox eliminate the need for plastic surgery?

This is a somewhat difficult question to answer. It is certain that Botox treatments at any age can greatly improve your appearance, but there are a number of things Botox can't do, such as remove spots and blemishes caused by sun damage or fill in sunken areas where your natural collagen and fat have disappeared.

Many physicians, we among them, believe that beginning Botox fairly early in life can indefinitely postpone many of the unsightly changes of aging, including most (but not all) wrinkles, a stringy neck, and some of the facial sagging caused by gravity and loss of natural padding. Even so, as you age, certain changes will appear, such as liver spots and other skin blemishes, which can benefit from other kinds of treatments. For more information on other rejuvenation treatments, see chapter 8.

For certain conditions, such as severely drooping eyelids or baggy eyes, plastic surgery is the only treatment that works. But for this as well as many other conditions, the use of Botox can put off plastic surgery for many years and improve upon its results afterward. For more information on combining Botox with other treatments, see chapter 8.

Will my wrinkles be worse than ever after Botox wears off?

This is a common and completely untrue myth about Botox. The truth is that as Botox gradually wears off, your wrinkles will gradually return. They won't be any worse than they were originally, and in fact may be less noticeable because you have gotten out of the habit of continually contracting the muscles in that area.

There is some evidence, though no conclusive proof, that using Botox before problems appear can delay severe wrinkling indefinitely. For a full discussion of this topic, see chapter 9.

Can I get financing for Botox treatments?

According to the web site ienhance.com, 29 percent of all Americans have considered having cosmetic surgery, and 60 percent of those people would have the procedure right away if they could get financing.

Since Botox is not covered for cosmetic purposes by insurance, financing could be a problem. However, financing for the specific purpose of cosmetic procedures is becoming more available in various places, including through many doctors' offices. Ienhance.com itself offers patient financing over the Internet. (For more information, see the list of web sites in Appendix A.)

Can I do anything to make the effect of my Botox injections last longer?

Unfortunately, the Botox injections will only last until the affected muscle or muscles grow new nerve endings and begin functioning again. However, there's a great deal you can do to keep your skin looking its best, including avoiding the sun, applying sunblock diligently, and using an anti–free radical serum or cream (such as topical vitamin C and E) and green tea extract (see our web site, InstituteBeaute.com). Using a prescription skin preparation such as Renova will help slow and even reverse aging and sun-induced changes. For more tips on keeping your complexion at its youthful best, see chapter 9.

Appendix A

Resources and Web Sites for More Information and Help in Locating a Physician

Botox Information Site

http://hometown.aol.com/drgulevich/myhomepage/business.html

This informative web site, maintained by Dr. Steven Gulevich, a Colorado neurologist, offers excellent information on the medical and cosmetic uses of Botox.

Yes They're Fake!

http://www.yestheyrefake.net/index.html

One of the most informative sites on the web, Yes They're Fake, maintained by a woman who has had multiple cosmetic procedures, serves as a kind of clearinghouse for all varieties of cosmetic procedures from creams to surgery. Marianne, the site's proprietor, has pulled together a variety of medical and lay sources as well as her own experience with the products and procedures she has tried. The site also includes chats and bulletin boards. Highly recommended. Direct link to the main Botox section:

http://www.yestheyrefake.net/botox.htm.

American Society of Aesthetic and Plastic Surgeons
http://surgery.org/default.htm

This site, home of the American Society of Aesthetic and Plastic Surgeons, offers extensive consumer advice on all aspects of cosmetic enhancement, including up-to-date information on all procedures as well as a search engine for locating a plastic surgeon in your area.

ienhance.com
http://www.ienhance.com

This web site, sponsored by iEnhance, a web-based community of patients, health care providers, and suppliers, offers a wide range of information on all aspects of aesthetic treatments, including a locator service for aesthetic physicians by area.

TMJ Disorders and Botox
http://www.max-facial.com/index.htm

Canadian doctors Marvin Schwarz and Brian Freund have been conducting ongoing studies on the use of Botox to treat temporomandibular joint (TMJ) disorders. For more information, check out their very informative web site.

Cerebral Palsy and Botox
http://www.ccmckids.org/departments/Orthopaedics/orthoed18.htm.

The Connecticut Children's Medical Center has a good fact page on cerebral palsy and Botox, including contact information for patients' families and doctors.

The Dystonia Foundation

http://www.dystonia-foundation.org/

The Dystonia Foundation maintains this web site, which offers a great deal of information on the various forms of dystonia and its treatments. For a direct link to a page explaining "The Botox Advantage," a program offered by Botox maker Allergan to help patients get insurance reimbursement for medical Botox treatments, click on this link:

http://www.dystonia-foundation.org/nsda/treatment/reimburse.asp

Institute Beauté

http://www.institutebeaute.com

The Institute Beauté website maintained by Dr. Everett M. Lautin and Dr. Suzanne M. Levine offers insight into noninvasive and minimally invasive rejuvenation treatments from head to toe.

Appendix B

Professional Articles

Alo, Kenneth M., et al. Botulinum toxin in the treatment of myofascial pain. *Clinic* 1997 (10:2);107–116.

Biddle, Jeff E., and Hamermesh, Daniel S. Beauty, productivity and discrimination: lawyers' looks and lucre. *J. Labor Economics* 1998 Jan (16:1):172–201.

Binder, William J., Blitzer, Andrew, and Brin, Mitchell F. Treatment of hyperfunctional lines of the face with Botulinum toxin A. *Dermatol. Surg.* 1998;24(11):1198–1205.

Brandt, F. S., and Bellman, B. Cosmetic use of botulinum A exotoxin for the aging neck. *Dermatol. Surg.* 1998 Nov;24(11):1232–1234.

Callaway, James E., Arezzo, Joseph C., and Grethlein, Andrew J. Botulinum toxin type A: an overview of its biochemistry and preclinical pharmacology. *Seminars in Cutaneous Med. and Surg.* 2001 Jun;20(2):127–136.

Carruthers, J. D. A., and Carruthers, A. Botulinum toxin and laser resurfacing for lines around the eyes. In Blitzer et al. (eds.), *Management of Facial Lines and Wrinkles*. Philadelphia: Lippincott Williams & Wilkins, 2000:303–313.

Foster, Larry; Clapp, Larry; Erickson, Marleigh; and Jabbari, Bahman. Botulinum toxin A and chronic low back pain. *Neurology* 56 2001 May; 1290–1293.

Hamermesh, Daniel S., and Biddle, Jeff E., Beauty and the labor market. *Amer. Econ. Rev.* 1994 Dec (84:5);1174–1194.

Naumann, M.; Hofmann, U.; Bergmann, I.; Hamm, H.; Toyka, K.; and Reiners, K. Focal hyperhidrosis: effective treatment with intracutaneous botulinum toxin. *Arch. Dermatol.* 1998 Mar;134:301–304.

Naver, H.; Swartling, C.; and Aquilonius, S. M. Treatment of focal hyperhidrosis with Botulinum toxin type A. Brief overview of methodology and 2 years' experience. *Eur. J. of Neurology* 1999;6(Suppl. 4):S117–S120.

Saadia, D., Voustianiouk, A., et al. Botulinum toxin type A in primary palmar hyperhidrosis. Randomized, single-blind, two-dose study. *Neurology* 2001;57:2095–2099.

Silberstein, Stephen, et al. Botulinum toxin type A as a migraine preventive treatment. *Headache* 2000;40:445–450.

Spencer, James M. Cosmetic uses of Botulinum toxin type B. *Cosm. Dermat.* 2002 Feb;15(2):11–14.

West, T. B., and Alster, T. S. Effect of Botlinum toxin type A on movement-associated rhytides following CO_2 resurfacing. *Dermatol. Surg.* 1999 April(25):259–261.

About the Authors

Everett M. Lautin, M.D., a graduate of Columbia College and Downstate College of Medicine, State University of New York (SUNY), former professor at the Albert Einstein College of Medicine, has been practicing medicine for more than twenty years. Dr. Lautin frequently lectures throughout the United States on nonsurgical plastic surgery and has been interviewed on this subject for articles in *Vogue, Glamour, New York* magazine, the *Times* magazine (London), and the *New York Times*. He lives in New York City. This is his first trade book.

Suzanne Levine, D.P.M., a graduate of Columbia University and New York College of Podiatric Medicine, has been practicing podiatry for more than twenty years. Dr. Levine is the author of five books, including *Your Feet Don't Have to Hurt, My Feet Are Killing Me,* and *50 Ways to Ease Foot Pain.* Dr. Levine is frequently interviewed for articles in such publications as *US Weekly, Elle, Glamour, Woman's Day, Vogue, W, Shape, Allure, Newsweek, Family Circle, Ladies Home Journal, New York* magazine, *USA Today,* the *New York Post,* and the *Wall Street Journal.* She is also a familiar presence on television and has appeared on *Today, The View, Weekend, Fox and Friends, The Oprah Winfrey Show,* and *Live with Regis and Kathie Lee.*

Drs. Everett Lautin and Suzanne Levine are the physician-owners of Institute Beauté (http://www.institutebeaute.com), a medical center on New York's Park Avenue, which provides head-to-toe rejuvenating medical treatments.